BREATHE

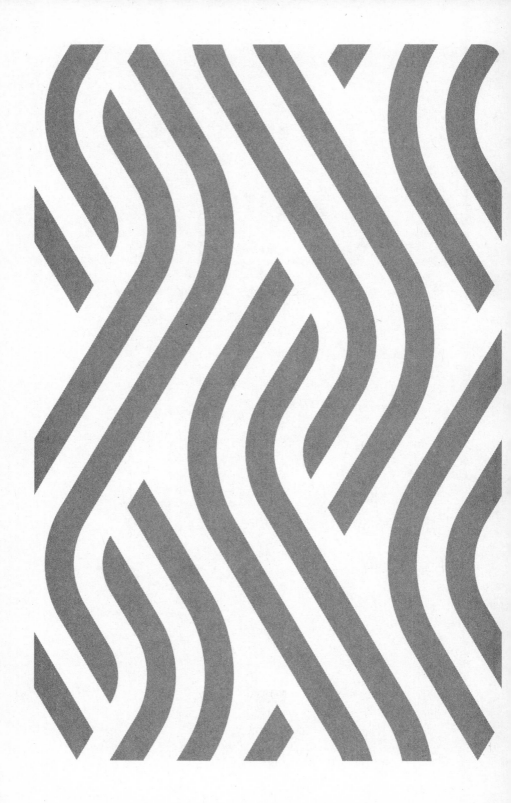

BREATHE

A LIFE IN FLOW

RICKSON GRACIE

with PETER MAGUIRE

DEY ST.
An Imprint of WILLIAM MORROW

DEY ST.

BREATHE. Copyright © 2021 by Rickson Gracie. All rights reserved. Printed in the United States of America. No part of this book may be used or reproduced in any manner whatsoever without written permission except in the case of brief quotations embodied in critical articles and reviews. For information, address HarperCollins Publishers, 195 Broadway, New York, NY 10007.

HarperCollins books may be purchased for educational, business, or sales promotional use. For information, please email the Special Markets Department at SPsales@harpercollins.com.

FIRST EDITION

Designed by Angela Boutin
Waves illustration © Jan/stock.adobe.com

Library of Congress Cataloging-in-Publication Data has been applied for.

ISBN 978-0-06-301895-2

21 22 23 24 25   LSC   10 9 8 7 6 5 4 3 2 1

To Hélio and Rockson Gracie,
who changed my view of life

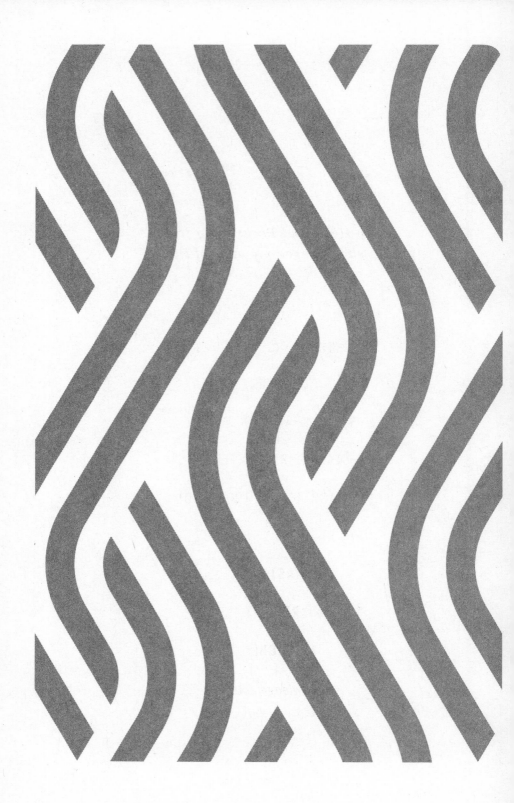

CONTENTS

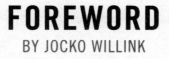

FOREWORD

BY JOCKO WILLINK

I WAS INTRODUCED TO JIU JITSU FOR THE FIRST TIME IN 1992 AS a young SEAL, fresh out of Basic Underwater Demolition/ SEAL (BUD/S) training, serving in a platoon at SEAL Team One. During our morning muster, a salty old master chief stopped by to talk to us. He was older than anyone I knew— although he was probably only a hair over forty—and years younger than I am today. But at the time, he seemed ancient.

"Does anyone want to learn how to fight?" he asked.

I wasn't expecting that at all, but I knew my answer immediately. *Of course I do!* I raised my hand along with a few other new guys.

While the SEAL teams now have programmatic combatives in the training pipeline, back in the early 1990s we learned next to nothing—some basic strikes, a hip throw or two, maybe a few self-defense moves against a highly telegraphed punch or kick. But it certainly didn't seem as if these choreographed moves would be effective in a real fight or combat situation.

"All right then, you guys with your hands up," said the master chief, "meet me at the Quonset hut by the gym at 1630."

Part of me thought, *What can this old man know?* I was young, strong, healthy, and highly motivated. He was just a lanky old man. I soon found out what he knew. He had a superpower. He knew Jiu Jitsu.

We showed up at the Quonset hut at the appointed time. Inside, there were mats on the ground. "All right. Take off your shoes and line up over there," he said, pointing to the wall. We followed his directions, and already I could feel my confidence melting away. "Take a seat. Now, one a time, attack me. When you have had enough, tap the mat or tap me three times." After saying that, he simply lay down on the floor. One of the guys stood up, walked over, and lunged at the master chief. Then, somehow, by some mysterious force, the young SEAL was reversed, the master chief had a hold on his neck, and the young SEAL tapped frantically. The master chief sprawled out on the ground again. "Who's next?"

I figured I would go. I stood up and walked over. I wouldn't make the mistake of my previous teammate, who rushed in. I would take my time, be smarter, more measured in my approach. The master chief did not seem concerned. After some grappling, I tried to grab his leg, and as soon as I did, he wrapped me up, twisted me around, isolated my arm, and straightened it out to the breaking point, at which time I tapped immediately.

This went on for almost an hour. Victim after victim, the master chief forced us to submit over and over again. Finally, when we were sweating, breathing hard, and too tired to keep trying, he looked at us and said, "Welcome to Gracie Jiu Jitsu."

The master chief, a SEAL by the name of Steve Bailey, had been training with the Gracie family in their garage in Torrance, California, for a little over a year. "And I'm just a white belt," he had said. I didn't know much about martial arts, but I knew that a white belt was just a beginner— *and he had mopped the floor with us.* I couldn't fathom what a black belt would be able to do. I also knew something else: I needed to learn this thing called Jiu Jitsu.

A few months later, the first Ultimate Fighting Championship took place in Denver, Colorado. Some people were wondering who would win. But my small group of friends, who were beginning to understand the power of Jiu Jitsu, knew who would win: the skinny Brazilian guy with the last name Gracie. That skinny guy was Royce Gracie, the first Ultimate Fighting Champion.

That is how my journey in Jiu Jitsu began. I eventually started training in San Diego with a Brazilian Jiu Jitsu black-belt instructor named Fábio Santos. As I tried to understand the history and philosophies and the hierarchies of the Jiu Jitsu world, I heard one name that would come up over and over again. The champion of the Gracie family. The undefeated fighter. The pinnacle of technique. The undisputed master of all things Jiu Jitsu.

Rickson Gracie.

There were stories of Rickson fighting in the streets of Rio de Janeiro to defend the honor of the Gracie name. Tales of his competition glory. Legends of his prowess on the mats. An unstoppable force who psychologically defeats his opponents before the fight even starts. Simply put, Rickson Gracie was the supreme master of Jiu Jitsu.

Of course, I was intrigued and inspired to seek out this legend. And luckily for me, my Jiu Jitsu instructor knew Rickson. In fact, he had trained under Rickson's brother Rolls and eventually was awarded his black belt by Rickson himself. I was also lucky because I lived and trained in San Diego, and Rickson's academy was just a couple of hours north, in Los Angeles.

I got permission from the navy for some time to go and train, and so I rented a cheap hotel room and showed up for classes at Rickson Gracie's studio on Pico Boulevard. At the time, Rickson was in the middle of his professional fighting career, so he did not teach the initial classes when I arrived. But his instructors had learned from the source, the master, and this was obvious from the detailed explanations and coaching they gave.

After four days of training, I showed up at the academy for another class, but something was different this time around. There had been ten to fifteen people in previous classes, but all of a sudden the studio was completely packed. I suspected what was happening, and my suspicions were confirmed when I heard chatter from the group: "Rickson is teaching tonight."

We all put on our gis and got on the mats. We started warming up and making small talk in idle anticipation for class to begin. Then, it happened: Rickson walked in. The entire place went silent. One of the subordinate instructors told us to circle up and started directing some exercises. I have never seen Jiu Jitsu students do jumping jacks, push-ups, and stretching with such intent. Finally, Rickson nodded at the subordinate instructor, who stopped the exercises and sat us down in a circle around the perimeter of the mat. Rickson walked out into the center of the circle and knelt comfortably on his knees. You could hear a pin drop. He sat for a period of time and then spoke in a soft but confident tone.

He talked about Jiu Jitsu. About offense and defense. About weight distribution and pressure. About leverage and patience and timing. He explained details and connected elements and clarified principles. I listened intently. We all did. Eventually, he taught some moves. They were basic, sure, but his granular instruction was something I had never experienced. We students paired up to try the moves while Rickson walked around and made adjustments: "More weight there," or "too much space," or "Not enough pressure."

After an hour, the instruction part of the class was over. It was time to spar—to engage in full-force training against other members of the class. My instructor from San Diego had told Rickson I was visiting his academy and asked if he would spar with me. Rickson approached me and asked if I wanted to train with him. "Yes, sir!"

At this time I was a blue belt in Jiu Jitsu, a lean 225 pounds. I worked out every day and had been training Jiu Jitsu hard for about two years. I had competed at the blue-belt level and won many competitions. I trained daily in San Diego with Dean Lister, a future world champion, and with many other highly skilled Jiu Jitsu practitioners. I was focused and motivated and determined.

None of those things mattered.

Rickson, who was forty pounds lighter than me, made me feel like a child.

He effortlessly controlled my movement, isolated my limbs, and submitted me over and over and over again. I fought hard, applied technique after technique, made adjustments, tried to surprise him, and used all the strength and trickery and skill and effort I could muster.

My resistance was futile.

There was nothing I could do.

Nothing.

When he was bored with my pitiful attempts at survival, we stopped sparring and talked for a bit. He asked me about SEAL training. He related to the warrior culture of my occupation. He also gave me an assessment of my Jiu Jitsu: "You do a good job staying calm in bad positions. That is an important thing."

Soon the class was over. We shook hands, and I thanked Rickson for his time and for his knowledge.

Over the next few days, I thought about what he had told me. "You do a good job staying calm in bad positions. That is an important thing." I realized that this did not apply only to Jiu Jitsu. It applied to my job in the SEAL teams as well. You are going to get put in bad positions. The enemy might get the upper hand. You might be outnumbered or outgunned. Panic will destroy you. *You have to stay calm.*

And that was only the beginning of the correlation I began to see from Jiu Jitsu to combat to leadership to business—to life itself. As I continued to learn Jiu Jitsu and progress in my SEAL career, Jiu Jitsu taught me much, but it was Rickson's words that initiated my journey. The principles of Jiu Jitsu can be applied to every endeavor in life.

You have stay calm when you are in bad situations.

You need to cover and conceal your intent with other maneuvers.

You need to utilize the simplest and most efficient methods.

You need to prioritize your focus of effort.

You need to train until you trust yourself to move intuitively, without having to think.

You need to move at the right time.

You have to defend critical areas.

You should not attack your enemy's strongpoints.

You must utilize leverage.

You cannot let your emotions drive your decisions.

You have to establish a good base foundation to build upon.

You cannot be overly aggressive, but you can't just allow things to happen.

When you make a move, you have to believe in what you are doing.

You have to be mentally strong.

You have to keep an open mind.

You have to continuously learn new techniques while always reinforcing the fundamentals.

You have to adapt your plan if circumstances change.

The list goes on and on and on.

When I deployed to Iraq as a SEAL combat leader, I continuously operated with these fundamental principles in my head, ones that I had understood because of Jiu Jitsu. I continue to utilize these principles now in the civilian world as well—as a businessman, a teacher, a father, and a coach. Jiu Jitsu gives me confidence but also humility, strength but also compassion, a disciplined code but also a free and open mind. As Rickson says, Jiu Jitsu is not just a sport; Jiu Jitsu is a philosophy, and it is at the root of everything we do.

Jiu Jitsu is a bond that connects people, and I am honored to be connected with Rickson and with many other superb Jiu Jitsu practitioners around the world. It is an honor for me to be asked to write the foreword to this book, not only because of what Rickson taught me about Jiu Jitsu, but also because of what Rickson and Jiu Jitsu taught me about life. This book furthers those lessons and reminds us of their staying power. Overcoming fear. Dealing with loss. Courage. Meaning. Strength. Honor. Pride. Forgiveness. The warrior way.

Enjoy this book. Learn from it. And go train Jiu Jitsu.

But most of all: Thank you, Rickson, for what you have done for Jiu Jitsu, for the world, and for me.

I will do my best to continue to represent this warrior tradition with honor.

Jocko Willink
October 2020

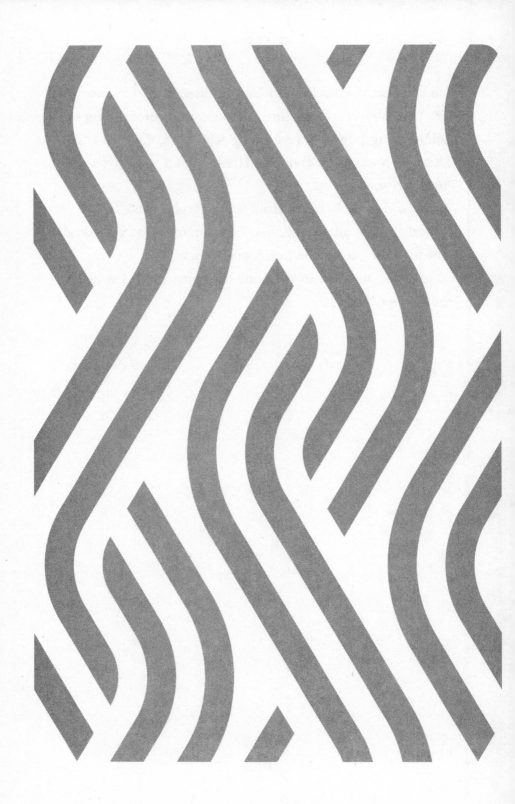

BREATHE

THE GRACIE CLAN

COME FROM A LONG LINE OF PROUD AND PUGNACIOUS PEOPLE
that I can trace back to Scotland, home of one of the world's
great warrior cultures. The Romans invaded Scotland (Cale-
donia) several times in the first three centuries AD, but the
fiercely independent clans fought back with a fury that impressed even the mighty legions. When there were no Romans or British left to fight, the clans fought each other.
Their leaders were willing to lead from the front and die in
the face of overwhelming odds and certain defeat.

Even though I grew up centuries later and a continent
away, these values were not too different from the ones that

my family lived by and tried to pass on to me, my brothers, and my cousins. Like our Scottish ancestors, it was only through fighting that one became a respected member of the Gracie clan. If one fought especially well, as I did, you became a favorite son, and after your martial arts odyssey, a respected leader.

Gracies began to leave Dumfries, Scotland, in the 1700s to seek their fortunes in the Americas. My distant relative Archibald Gracie filled a ship with precious cargo, sailed it to New York City, made a small fortune, and started a shipping business with American founding father Alexander Hamilton.

Gracie Mansion, Archibald Gracie's country house on New York City's East River, sounded to me like a colonial American version of my family's ranch in Teresópolis, Brazil. It was a place where future American presidents, titans of commerce, and European dignitaries gathered on the weekends to relax and escape the heat and squalor of the city. Since 1942 it has served as the home of New York City's mayors.

Archibald's son, Archibald Jr., was a very successful New York merchant, but his grandson Archibald III was a warrior. At West Point, he earned superintendent Robert E. Lee's respect after he got beaten up in a fight on the parade grounds. When Gracie was called into Lee's office, he refused to give up the name of the man he was fighting. After his opponent turned himself in, Lee did not punish either of them.

When America's Civil War broke out, Archibald Gracie III

sided with the Confederacy. He started the war as a major, but after fighting heroically in some of the conflict's fiercest battles, Gracie was a brigadier general at the age of twenty-nine. During the siege of Petersburg, Virginia, in 1864, he constructed the Gracie Salient, a defensive masterpiece full of trenches, bunkers, obstacles, and mortar pits designed to keep the Union Army at bay.

During the nine-month siege of Petersburg, Robert E. Lee came to inspect Gracie's position. It was only a few hundred yards away from the Union lines, and when Lee tried to peek over the wall to survey the enemy soldiers, Gracie climbed up onto the wall and stood like a human shield in front of the astonished commander of the Confederate Army. "Why, Gracie, you will certainly be killed," said Lee.

"It is better, General, that I be killed than you. When you get down, I will."

Robert E. Lee survived the Civil War, but Archibald Gracie III did not. When Lee received the news that Gracie had been killed by a mortar shell at Petersburg, he wrote, "It was a great grief to me. I do not know how to replace him."

The Brazilian side of the Gracie family was also full of bold and dynamic people. My great-great-grandfather, George Gracie, left Dumfries and arrived in Rio de Janeiro in 1826. Initially, he worked in the import-export business, but he married into an upper-class Brazilian family and became a director at the Bank of Brazil. His son, my great-grandfather Pedro, also became a prominent banker.

Pedro's son, my grandfather Gastão Gracie, was educated in Germany, where he received a degree in chemistry. After he finished his education in Europe, Gastão moved to the port city of Belém, Brazil, near the mouth of the Amazon River. Although he was trained to be a diplomat, my grandfather's nature was anything but diplomatic. He had a bad temper, was impulsive, and spent money faster than he could make it. Too late to cash in on the rubber boom, he gambled, manufactured dynamite, and managed a circus instead.

The American Circus brought fighters from all over the world for bouts with Brazilian challengers in Belém. One of those who made his way to Amazonia was a Japanese fighter named Hideyo Maeda. Trained in both traditional Jiu Jitsu and the more sporting art of Judo, Maeda was one of Japan's greatest judokas before he became a prize fighter. Traditional Japanese Jiu Jitsu was developed for armed combat on the battlefield, but Judo was created in the late 1880s by Jigarō Kanō as a safer, more sporting, weaponless alternative.

Maeda left Japan in 1904 to conduct public Judo demonstrations in the United States at Columbia University, Princeton, and West Point. Afterwards, he remained in America, where he fought and won prize fights in Georgia, North Carolina, and Alabama before moving on to fight in Europe. Fighting under the name Conde Koma, or Count Combat, Maeda won hundreds of bouts against boxers, champion wrestlers, and giant brawlers all over the world. By the time he settled in Brazil, he had been outside Japan for a decade and would never return.

The necessities of real fighting forced the Japanese fighter to modify his traditional Judo and Jiu Jitsu techniques in order to make them more effective. Maeda fought both grappling matches and no-holds-barred fights that were called *vale tudo* ("anything goes") in Brazil. Much closer to a street fight than modern MMA, in *vale tudo* there were no gloves, no weight divisions, and no time limits. A small fighter like Maeda, often heavily outweighed by his opponents, had to adopt a strategic and patient approach to fighting.

In 1917, my grandfather, Gastão Gracie, took his fifteen-year-old son Carlos to watch a fight at Belém's Theatro da Paz. Because of his blond hair and bright blue eyes, people called my uncle Carlos the Little Gringo, and according to my family, he was hyperactive and always in trouble. After Carlos watched the five-four, 145-pound Japanese man control and dominate much larger opponents, he had a revelation: a fighter who used technique, strategy, and intelligence could defeat a fighter who had only size and strength.

Maeda settled in Belém with his wife and daughter. Gastão introduced him to some of the region's leaders and helped him get land for Japanese immigrants to build farms in the rain forest. Maeda opened a martial arts school in Belém, where he and an assistant taught my uncles Carlos, Oswaldo, George, Gastão Jr., and a handful of others his modified style of Jiu Jitsu.

After Gastão Gracie went bankrupt in the 1920s, the brothers moved to Rio and opened their first Jiu Jitsu academy. They were confident enough in their abilities to invite fighters from any style to test their skills in a match against

Jiu Jitsu. A "Gracie challenge" could be a sporting match that a tap on the ground could end at any time, but my uncles also fought *vale tudo* matches. Because my father, Hélio, was the youngest of the brothers, Carlos was almost a father figure to him. My father would later say that he owed his life to Uncle Carlos because he educated him and gave him a set of philosophical principles to live by.

When all of your brothers are fighters, there are bound to be fights. Even though the Gracies would close ranks against outsiders, there was always tension between family members that sometimes boiled over. While Hélio followed his eldest brother's orders like gospel, Uncle George "the Red Cat" Gracie had his own ideas. George was an excellent fighter and the most athletic of the brothers. But he was also a bohemian who liked to gamble and party, which meant he was often at odds with his more austere older brother, Carlos. Eventually the brothers went their separate ways, and the only one who stuck with Carlos through thick and thin was my father, Hélio. Some said that their relationship was so close that they were like a finger and its nail.

My father was far from the best athlete in the family. When he was a child, a doctor told him not to exercise because of his vertigo. My dad used to say, "I was born weak, I'll die weak. I pass for strong because of Jiu Jitsu." Because Hélio did not have the option of using power, he had to rely on leverage, sensitivity, and timing to compensate for his lack of strength. I know this might sound like an exaggeration, but Hélio Gracie was to Jiu Jitsu what Albert Einstein was to physics. He greatly improved the martial art by further developing a position called the guard that was both defensive and offensive, which allowed him to fight off his back with his opponent between his legs. Not only was he able to defend himself from punches, but he could also control and submit his opponents with an arsenal of chokes and joint locks. Although the position had existed previously in Judo, because of my dad's size and the violent nature of *vale tudo* fights, he modified and modernized it.

Slight and physically unimposing, Hélio Gracie was a perfect poster child for a martial art that claimed to be the triumph of intelligence over brute strength. An early commercial for Gracie Jiu Jitsu featured a skinny guy with an attractive woman on a Rio beach. In it, a muscle-bound bully slaps the skinny guy to the ground and leaves with his girlfriend. In the next scene, the skinny guy is shown signing up for classes at the Gracie Academy, training in Jiu Jitsu, and then returning to the same beach a few weeks later to confront the bully. This time, he blocks the muscleman's punch, throws him to the ground, breaks his arm, and leaves with the girl. They really don't make commercials like they used to.

To Carlos Gracie, Jiu Jitsu was as much about psychology as it was about martial arts. He believed that because the martial art had cured his male insecurity and given him confidence and peace of mind, it could do the same for others. He used to say that he used Jiu Jitsu to turn chickens into stallions. My uncle Carlos was a very eccentric guy. He almost always wore white linen, walked around barefoot, and claimed that he had a direct, personal relationship with a benevolent spirit who gave him extrasensory perception (ESP). He often rose before dawn to meditate under the sun's first rays, and he sunbathed naked because he believed doing so would help him sire strong children. My uncle talked about biorhythms, nutrition, digestion, food combining, but rarely traditional religion. He believed that the letters R, K, and C were powerful ones, which is why so many of my family's names begin with them.

Carlos Gracie attracted a number of followers who shared his unique worldview. One of them was a prominent businessman named Oscar Santa Maria, who became his greatest patron. He helped Carlos invest his money and run his day-to-day affairs so that my uncle was free to devote all of his time to Gracie Jiu Jitsu. Their relationship got more complicated after Carlos married Oscar's fiancée and had three children with her. After three decades as his disciple, Santa Maria became my uncle's archenemy and sued him for fraud.

I believe that my uncle Carlos was deeply affected by two deaths that occurred early in his life. When he was a young man, a previous fiancée contracted typhoid and, while suffering from a very high fever, jumped out of a window to her death. Carlos was so distraught that he, too, considered suicide. A decade later, his first wife, Carmen, the mother of six of his children, got tuberculosis. When she went to a sanatorium, Carlos ignored the doctors' warnings about this highly contagious disease and moved into the sanatorium with her.

Although he exposed himself to the disease, he refused to leave her side until Carmen died in 1940. Miraculously, Carlos never contracted the disease.

After the two loves of his life died, Carlos Gracie decided to father as many children, preferably boys, as possible, and he encouraged my father to do the same. Their goal was to create a clan of fighters. Between 1932 and 1967, Carlos and Hélio fathered *thirty* children with *eight* different women; twenty-one of them were boys. When Margarida, my father's first wife, the woman I consider my mother, was unable to get pregnant, my uncle came up with a plan. My father, with my mother's knowledge and consent, would impregnate our African Brazilian babysitter, Belinha, who gave birth to me and my older brothers Rorion and Relson. The whole thing was an elaborate ruse. Margarida wore a fake belly during Belindha's pregnancies and when the time came for her to give birth, she went to the hospital and came home with a baby. Not even her best friends knew! When I was young and looked at myself in the mirror and saw my freckles, I thought they were from my Scottish blood. Little did I know that I was half African Brazilian!

My mother, Margarida, was a well-educated, upper-class girl whose father was a millionaire who owned a huge import/export company and lots of property. After she divorced her first husband, which was very uncommon in Brazil at that time, she fell madly in love with Hélio, who was a rough guy. Not only did she polish him, she also introduced him to Rio's high society. Even though Margarida was passionately in love with him, their relationship was one-sided. Hélio was ice cold and didn't care how anyone felt other than my uncle Carlos. He was old-fashioned Brazilian macho and believed that women belonged in the nursery and the kitchen. He even went so far as to say that he never loved a woman, because love was a manifestation of weakness, and that he had sex only for the sake of procreation. In his mind, his mission was bigger than these kinds of sensitivities.

Even though Carlos and Hélio were a team bound by their mission to create a clan of fighters, they had very different roles. When I was born, in 1958, Carlos was well into his fifties and played no role in my martial-arts training. He was our family's nutritionist and philosopher. My uncle was also responsible for the Gracie diet. Carlos believed disease was the body's form of protest, the way it told you that something was wrong with you. Food causes alkaline or acidic reactions in the blood, he told us, and he attempted to eliminate acidity. My father did not eat meat. While I grew up eating beef, chicken, and fish, we ate it in moderation. As important as what you eat is when you eat and what foods you combine together. Typically, Gracies would eat one starch, one protein, and then a salad. I would never eat rice and beans at the same time. Meals were spaced five hours apart to allow the body to absorb the nutrients from the food.

Sweets to us were not cookies and ice cream. They were papayas, mangoes, figs, or watermelon juice. Sugar, processed foods, alcohol, and coffee were all strictly prohibited. I grew up thinking that eating chocolate was like drinking rat poison! Coca-Cola? Poison! Cake and cookies? Poison! As kids, we were amazed by how much longer Uncle Carlos took to finish his meals; he would chew each bite for over a minute, and it would take him more than an hour to eat a small plate of food.

If Carlos Gracie was our philosopher, Hélio Gracie was our general. We were all supposed to fight, eat, and have courage like him, and this was no small feat. Even though my uncle's values were spiritual and metaphysical, my father's were closer to those of the samurai. Both my dad and uncle believed in reincarnation, and Hélio thought that he had been a Japanese warrior in a previous life. Once, a spiritual medium, who claimed she could see past lives, came to our ranch with a family friend to pay a social visit. When the medium met my father, she began to cry in a series of convulsions and then said, "You were a bloody shogun in Japan!"

Hélio Gracie didn't just talk the talk. He was probably the bravest man I've ever met. In 1947, he and Carlos were traveling aboard a ship in the open ocean near the Abrolhos Islands. The sun was starting to set when someone screamed, "Man overboard!" The captain stopped the ship, and crew members manned a lifeboat and lowered it into the stormy sea. When the lifeboat reached the drowning man, they could not get him into the lifeboat without the risk of capsizing it. After a couple of halfhearted attempts, the crew got scared, began to row back to the ship, and left the man to drown. My father and uncle were watching the tragedy unfold from the deck, and when my father saw the lifeboat

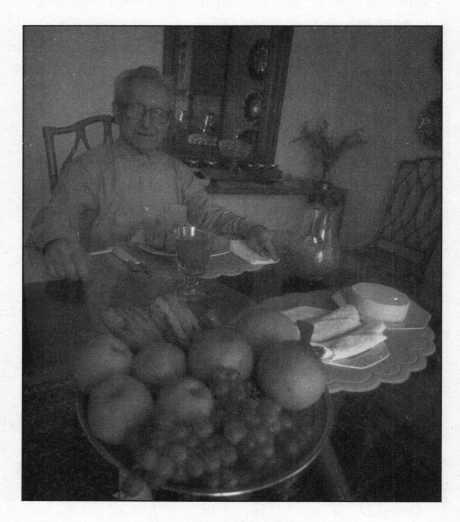

CARLOS GRACIE, RIO DE JANEIRO, 1988.
PHOTOGRAPH COURTESY OF MARCOS PRADO / @REVISTATRIP, 1988.

returning to the ship, he turned to my uncle and said, "Fuck! They're going to let him die!" Hélio stripped off his clothes, dived into the sea in his underwear, and as he swam past the lifeboat he yelled, "Go back!" The lifeboat turned around and began to follow him back to the drowning man.

My dad was able to lift the victim out of the water so the crew could drag him into their boat. By now it was getting dark and one of the lifeboat crew members began to panic and said, "We're not going to make it back to the ship!" Before the panic could spread, my father took the man's oar and said, "C'mon guys! Let's row back to the ship!" This decisiveness and confidence settled the crew. By the time they made it back, conditions were so bad that it took almost an hour to hoist the lifeboat back on deck. If my father had not imposed his strong and confident mind-set on the lifeboat crew, the panic would have spread like wildfire.

Emotions are contagious. Hélio used to say that you had to break the emotional wave before it broke on you. Take a car salesman for example. When you walk onto the lot, he intercepts you and comes with a pitch: "You can drive off this lot in this new car today! No money down!" Of course, you want a new car and naturally you don't want to put any money down, but if you let the salesman gain momentum, he'll get you to agree to anything he wants. You can't allow yourself to be swept away by a wave without knowing where it is going to take you. Instead, when the salesman approaches, you say, "No, thank you," which breaks his momentum. Now he has to regroup. My dad believed that if your mind and will are not strong, you'll spend your entire life getting carried away by your desires and weaknesses. You'll spend your whole life paying for things you don't want.

By the time I was born, my father was already one of Brazil's biggest sports icons. In addition to being an incredibly tough fighter, he was also a showman of the highest order who publicly challenged boxing icons Primo Carnera, Joe Louis, and Ezzard Charles. Although the boxers all declined, in 1932 American wrestler Fred Ebert accepted seventeen-year-old Hélio's challenge. Ebert outweighed him by about fifty pounds, but they fought for an hour and forty minutes before the police stopped the fight. Two years later, my dad fought 225-pound world-champion wrestler Władek Zbyszko to a draw.

When Japan's greatest judoka, Masahiko Kimura, traveled to Brazil in 1951, Hélio also challenged him. Kimura agreed to fight my dad if he could first defeat Yukio Kato, one of the black belts traveling with him. My dad's first fight with Kato was declared a draw, but Hélio choked him unconscious in their rematch, clearing the way for a match with the Judo champion.

Hélio and Kimura squared off in front of twenty thousand spectators at Rio's Maracanãzinho Stadium a week later, and even the president of Brazil attended the match. The judoka outweighed my dad by eighty pounds and threw him around the ring like a rag doll but could not finish him. At one point, my dad went unconscious, but because he didn't tap, Kimura thought his choke wasn't working and released it, and Hélio regained consciousness. Thirteen minutes into the fight, the Judo champion secured a bent-arm lock, and again my dad refused to tap. Kimura kept twisting and ripping at his shoulder. Still, Hélio refused to tap, but Kimura kept cranking, and my uncle Carlos threw in the towel. My dad later said he got his samurai spirit from Kimura and named the bent-arm lock (*ude garami* in Judo) the kimura.

Hélio Gracie didn't fight for money or fame; he fought for the honor of the Gracie family. In 1955, when he was forty-four and retired from fighting, Waldemar "the Black Panther" Santana challenged him. The muscular African Brazilian marble cutter was sixteen years younger and sixty pounds heavier. Santana had been my dad's student and a friend and training partner of my cousin Carlson Gracie. He'd worked as the academy's locker-room attendant but quit after a dispute with Hélio.

My father and Santana agreed to a *vale tudo* match with no time limit at a YMCA in Rio. A big, raucous crowd watched them fight for three hours and forty-eight minutes. In the end, Santana knocked my father unconscious with a kick to the head. As in his 1951 loss to Kimura, Hélio conceded that Santana had beaten him in a fair fight, but he was proud of the fact that he never quit and never considered himself defeated. This became a very important distinction for Gracies. From a very young age, it was drilled into us that there was no shame in losing but there was shame in quitting or not fighting. Later that year, my cousin Carlson avenged my dad by defeating Santana at Maracanãzinho Stadium, becoming

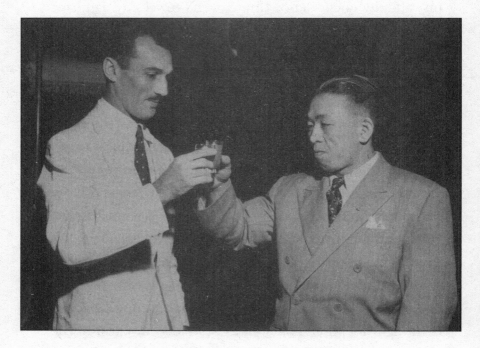
HÉLIO GRACIE AND YUKIO KATO SHARE A TOAST.
PHOTOGRAPH COURTESY OF THE RICKSON GRACIE COLLECTION.

the undisputed family champion and a new Brazilian sports hero.

My brothers, my cousins, and I wanted to follow in Hélio and Carlson's footsteps and carry our family's flag into battle. My father and uncle attempted to instill us with courage even as babies. One Gracie family tradition was to throw male babies into the air before their first birthday to build confidence and trust between father and son. The process is gradual. You start by just bouncing the baby in your hands. If he laughs, you bounce him a little higher. Next, you throw the baby a few inches in the air and let him fall back into your hands. Next, you throw him a foot in the air, and then another foot. My dad and uncle were able to play catch with some babies, like me and my brother Rolls. Not every Gracie baby rose to this challenge, and I believe that they used this as a test to determine which of us would be "game" fighters.

One of my earliest childhood memories is of a time when I was four and we were all at the beach at Copacabana. When the Gracies went to the beach, we didn't just build sand castles. My dad used to have us hold on to a tire inner tube and he'd tow us out to sea. Each time he took us a little farther out. One day he said, "C'mon, boys, today we will go see Christ." He towed us so far out into the ocean that we could see over the buildings that blocked the view of the hundred-foot-tall statue of Jesus that stands above Rio on Mount Corcovado more than a mile away in the Tijuca National Park. Just when we could see the Christ the Redeemer statue, the inner tube sprang a leak and began to

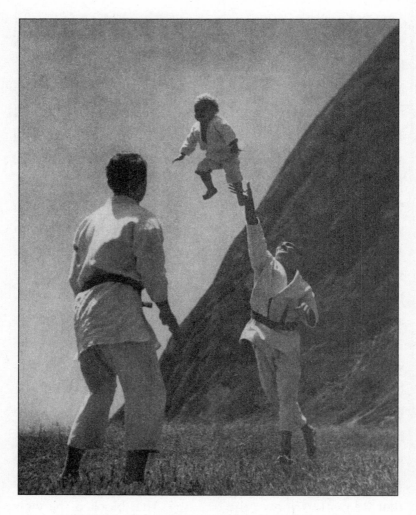

CARLOS AND HÉLIO GRACIE PLAY CATCH WITH ROLLS GRACIE.
PHOTOGRAPH COURTESY OF THE RICKSON GRACIE COLLECTION.

piss out all of its air. First, my dad calmed everyone down, put me on his back, and said, "OK, boys, we have to swim back in." Without a moment's hesitation, we all put our heads down, started swimming, and made it back to shore without a problem.

Even when facing death, my father remained composed. When I was five, we were driving in his Jeep on a piece of rural property that my mother inherited. Hélio now managed the property and had recently cut off water to some of the tenants because of a billing dispute. Suddenly, a VW van cut us off, my dad slammed on the brakes, and we slid to a stop that almost threw me out of the car. A Brazilian councilman, followed by his son and armed henchmen, jumped out and surrounded us. "You cut off my water!" the councilman said. "Now, you're going to die!" Outnumbered and outgunned, Hélio tried to talk them down and at one point grew quiet, expecting the worst. One of the goons shot at my dad but the bullet only grazed his earlobe. When Hélio fell to the ground, another guy shot him in the leg. I yelled, "Don't hurt my dad! Don't hurt my dad!" but they pushed me out of the way and smashed his face with the butt of a gun. I think they wanted to kill Hélio but didn't because I was there. "I thought you were tough!" the councilman said. "I can kill you anytime I want! If you don't stay out of our business, I will!" Then they got back into their van and drove off, leaving my dad bleeding in the dirt. I was upset, but my dad was totally calm. He put his arm around me and said, "Don't worry, son, everything's going to be OK." Even though the goons had threatened to kill my dad if he went to the police, after he got his wounds treated, Hélio went straight to the police station and reported the crime. In the end, he and the councilman reached an uneasy peace.

My dad was a tough and demanding teacher, but he never pushed us the way I see some parents push their kids in Jiu Jitsu today. Why would a kid want to train if his dad yells at him the whole time? My father understood this, and his message was always, "If you win, great! But if you don't, stand up and try again!" My earliest memories of Jiu Jitsu are fun, even playful. My father's academy in downtown Rio took up an entire floor at a fancy office building and resembled a country club more than a Jiu Jitsu academy. Each student had his own locker and received a clean gi and towel every time he trained.

The initial Gracie Jiu Jitsu curriculum consisted of forty self-defense classes that focused on empowering students. The goal was to prepare them mentally, physically, and psychologically for a physical confrontation and to build a foundation of confidence that would give them peace of mind. My dad's handpicked instructors taught a hundred private lessons a day to Brazil's business leaders and politicians. The tuition was expensive, most of the lessons were private, and Hélio kept his instructors on a very short leash. Not only did they have to follow a strict self-defense curriculum, but they were fined for every minute they were late.

Initially, we kids went to the academy just to play tug-of-war or have a game of soccer. We were introduced to Jiu Jitsu slowly, nothing like what I see these days. Today, too many parents push their kids to compete before they are ready. For young kids, Jiu Jitsu should be nothing more than a fun form of recreation that introduces them to the movements through games and structured play. As they get older, you can introduce more Jiu Jitsu, but it should be playful. If you push kids too hard, too young, they will quit forever. Parents should never burden their kids with their unfulfilled ambitions, frustrations, anxiety, or any other form of emotional baggage. The parents' support must be consistent. The most important thing is that the child gets the experience—win, lose, or draw—without judgment.

My first memory of competing in Jiu Jitsu isn't even about Jiu Jitsu or the fight itself. It's about the message my father sent me before my match, which has stuck with me for my entire life. Because I was only six, there was no division for me, so my dad put me in the bracket with the older kids. Right before I was about to step onto the mat to fight, he said, "Rickson, if you lose the fight, I'll give you two gifts. If you win the fight, I'll give you one." When I realized that my dad wouldn't be upset if I lost, the pressure melted away. I lost the match but didn't feel bad because my dad wasn't mad. Instead, he was proud of me for competing against the older kids. All I felt was approval. There was no blame or stress. Children who get involved in Jiu Jitsu at a young age learn to be more than just strong and competitive. Jiu Jitsu is much more fluid than Judo or Karate and requires patience, not just aggression, and forces students to develop strategies to find comfort in uncomfortable situations. This is where Jiu Jitsu differs from both wrestling and Judo.

Hélio always stressed the importance of sharpness, timing, and the killer instinct. He liked to tell us parables about fighting. God knows if they were even true, but we believed them. One of his favorites was about the Indians in the Brazilian rain forest who hunted jaguars with spears. He used it as a metaphor for the way we were supposed to use the *pisão*, or side kick, like a jab to intercept and keep an opponent at bay. When the Indian hunter spotted a jaguar in a tree, he would make noise in order to draw the animal's attention, act scared, and then allow the big cat to stalk him. The hunter was clever. He did not brandish his spear but kept it concealed instead. Jaguars are ambush predators. They leap onto the back of their prey and break its neck with a bite to the nape of the neck. The Indian would let the jaguar get within striking range but, just as it leaped to attack and was fully committed, would turn and drive his spear through the big cat's chest.

"You have to be like the Indian!" Hélio would say, "You have to have courage to allow him to think that he is in range to get you, then get him to commit and intercept him with the *pisão* the same way the Indian uses his spear." My dad would then make the point that blind courage, without timing and strategy, was not enough to kill a jaguar. Then he would relate it to fighting: "If a karate fighter wants to kick you in the face, first he has to get in range. If you can intercept his leg with a kick of your own, he can never get set to throw a kick. But, like the Indian, you have to believe in your ability to do it!"

Even as a small boy, I silently observed, from close proximity, fear, courage, aggression, and cowardice. I noticed small things about people because they provided clues about their true nature. Things as simple as the way someone shook my hand, the way people acted when they won, and the way they acted when they lost told me a lot. I often wondered why a guy who beat me so mercilessly made excuses not to train with my older brothers. I didn't judge them; I just knew that I didn't want to be like them.

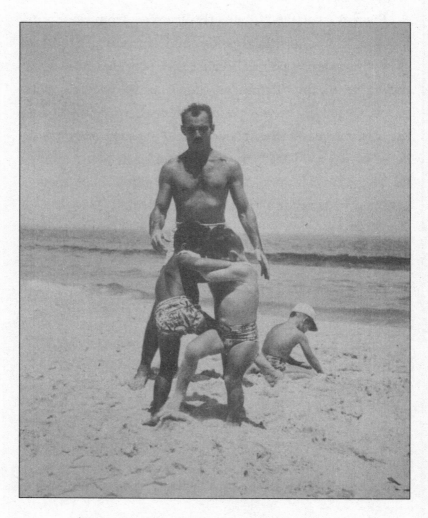

HÉLIO WATCHES RORION AND RELSON SPAR ON THE BEACH.
PHOTOGRAPH COURTESY OF THE RICKSON GRACIE COLLECTION.

GROWING UP GRACIE

I REALLY BEGAN TO UNDERSTAND HOW DIFFERENT MY FAMILY WAS at the age of seven when I went to school for the first time. I was shocked when my mother dropped me off and I saw my classmates clinging to their mothers' legs, crying, and pissing in their pants like babies. When the teacher asked us what we wanted to be when we grew up, the other students gave the usual answers: fireman, nurse, cop, teacher. When she got to me, I said without hesitation, "A fighter! A champion!" I wanted to be just like my dad.

When I brought my lunch of apples and whole-wheat bread to school, kids would beg to try it. "You can have a little taste," I'd tell them, "but that's all, because I don't want to eat your shit." When I went to another student's house after school and he opened their refrigerator, all I saw were boxes of packaged food. I didn't even know what it was. The only things in our refrigerator were carrots, radishes, apples, and fresh-squeezed juices. The only bread we ever ate was homemade wheat bread.

One day, a classmate was bragging that he had five brothers and sisters. I laughed and told him that my uncle had twenty-one kids and seven wives! My classmates didn't believe me, so I explained to them that some of the mothers left after the babies were born. Little did I know that my own birth mother was one of them! Although this seemed normal to me, I could see by the looks on my classmates' faces that it was not normal to them.

Even at seven years old, my worldview had already been shaped by Jiu Jitsu, my family's warrior ethos, and my brothers and cousins. If Hélio Gracie was the general, then my brothers and cousins were his colonels, captains, sergeants, and privates. The Gracies were a tough crowd. Every time we went to the movies, one of my cousins would always make sure to bring a big bill. When it was time to pay for the bus or a movie, he'd say, "You guys pay for me because I don't have change." One day we all rebelled and made my cousin pay for all of us. If one of my brothers knew that you were afraid of spiders, he would catch one, put it in a box, and then scare you with it. I learned at a young age to never lower my guard.

I studied all my brothers with great interest when we

trained because they had different strengths and weaknesses. I wanted to know: Who was brave? Who was scared? Who would fight to the death? Who was crazy? Who was indecisive? Nobody impressed me more than my brother Rolls. A decade older than me, he was our leader and my idol because he was an incredibly charismatic person and a natural warrior.

Rolls was Uncle Carlos's son from Claudia, an eighteen-year-old woman who worked for my family. Because my mother, Margarida, could not have children, Uncle Carlos gave Rolls to my dad to raise as his own son when he was a baby. Rolls grew up with us and shared a room with me for much of my childhood. Claudia moved to New York City to work for Lufthansa when my brother was around ten, one of the perks of the job being heavily discounted airline tickets. This enabled Rolls to travel all over the world before any of us. He learned to speak English, as well as Italian. Rolls felt as comfortable on Park Avenue as in the jazz clubs of Harlem.

My brother's open mind helped him in Jiu Jitsu because he was willing to look outside of it for ideas when other family members were not. Rolls trained and competed in Judo, wrestling, and Sambo, which he used to improve Jiu Jitsu. Like Hélio, he always wanted to win by submission and had an aggressive attacking style. If I disappointed Rolls, there was nothing that I was not willing to do to redeem myself. At thirteen, a big guy got me in a tight headlock. Instead of calmly defending my neck, I panicked, struggled, and eventually tapped out. I was embarrassed that I tapped while

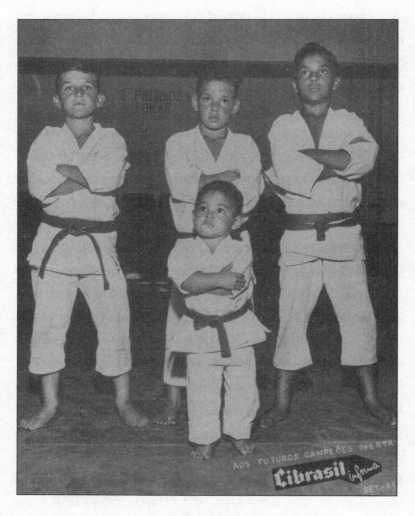

RICKSON GRACIE (FRONT CENTER) WITH HIS BROTHERS
ROLLS, RELSON, AND RORION.
PHOTOGRAPH COURTESY OF THE RICKSON GRACIE COLLECTION.

Rolls had watched. I got home and asked him to roll me up in the carpet for ten minutes and not to let me out no matter how loud I screamed or begged. It was summertime and very hot in Rio. The rug stank. During the first few minutes inside the carpet cocoon, I thought I might suffocate and die. Once I resigned myself to my fate and embraced the discomfort, my breathing slowed and I lost all sense of time. The next day my brother rolled me up for fifteen minutes, and by the end of the week I had conquered my fear.

This experience taught me an important lesson about Jiu Jitsu: sometimes it's not about escaping but about finding whatever comfort you can in hell. Something as small as turning my rib cage slightly so I can breathe a little easier can be the difference between victory and defeat. This was less a technical revelation to me than it was a mental one.

When Rolls taught me Jiu Jitsu or took me surfing, he was a generous teacher, but he also had a terrifying side, because he never considered consequences. I was twelve years old and home alone watching television when Rolls walked in with some friends and turned off the lights. He opened the window as his friend pulled an Uzi out of his bag and handed it to my brother, who started shooting it out the window. *Trrrrrr!!! Trrrrrr!!!* "This shit is good!" he said. Our apartment faced Guanabara Bay and the other side of the bay was a mile and a quarter away, so he was unlikely to hit anyone. Still, I was terrified watching Rolls laugh maniacally as the gun ejected spent brass. Next, we heard police sirens, and Rolls told everyone to hide on the floor. Even though the police eventually went away, I was scared because Brazil at that time was governed by the military dictatorship.

Rolls believed that the Brazilian dictatorship was wrong, and he had friends who were part of the leftist insurgency. During the 1960s, a Marxist group called the Ação Libertadora Nacional (National Liberation Action), or ALN, carried out a campaign of bombings and kidnappings in Brazil. The ALN accused the dictatorship of selling the nation to the US government and American multinational corporations. After ALN members kidnapped the West German and American ambassadors and ransomed them for the release of political prisoners, the dictatorship's Department of Social and Political Order (DOPS) really began to crack down. This federal police agency began to arrest, torture, and sometimes kill anyone they suspected of collaborating with the ALN.

Rolls's friend Rico was a member of the ALN and was rarely without a bag full of guns and grenades. Although Rolls was not a member, he read their leftist literature and was sympathetic to their cause. The Department of Social and Political Order suspected that my brother and my older cousin Robson were revolutionaries and arrested them. Robson's fighting career was over by then, and he had become an outspoken, street-smart guy.

I was twelve or thirteen and at home with my mom and dad when there was an unexpected knock on the door. My dad opened it and two federal police officers were standing in front of him. "With all due respect, Mr. Gracie," one said, "your son told us that there is a military weapon in your house. We've come to get it."

At first, my dad said that there were no guns in his house. Then the policeman said, "We believe you, Mr. Gracie, but you need to be absolutely sure. There will be big problems for your son if he is lying about this."

Then my dad told the officers to wait on the couch and turned to me and said, "Rickson, go into your brother's room and see if you can find the gun." I went into Rolls's room and began to go through his things and found a big black rifle in the back of his closet. It was an FN FAL, the official rifle of the Brazilian military.

I brought the gun out to the living room and handed it to the policeman, who said, "That is what we were looking for." Although Rolls was stripped and photographed after his arrest, he was released the same day.

When my brother got home, he looked shaken. "Man, Rolls! If you're not careful," Hélio warned him, "you won't just lose your career; you'll lose your life!" Even though my dad had many important political and military connections, the Department of Political and Social Order officers were a law unto themselves. Dad continued, "We have no control over these people. They do whatever they want. There are motherfuckers on the right and motherfuckers on the left. Politics is not for us."

Rolls apologized and promised that he would never get involved in politics again. Robson, on the other hand, was not so lucky. He was tortured and interrogated for two months straight. When he was finally released, he was a shell of his former self for a while. Rolls's friend Rico was even more unlucky. He was eventually captured, tortured, and killed.

Nine years older than me, my brother Rorion could not have been more different from Rolls. Hélio's first son with our birth mother Belindha, Rorion was ten months younger than Rolls. Rorion had an easygoing nature, and while he was never the fighter that Rolls was, he was a born teacher. Training with Rorion included the theory behind such concepts as positioning, technique, leverage, and base. He explained Jiu Jitsu much better than Rolls, who was impatient and saw things as either black or white. He had a big influence on my teaching style and got me to focus as much on the person as the techniques. Our father taught us that a good teacher taught the techniques well, but that a great teacher taught what each individual student needed to learn, in strife or in life. Rorion was a great teacher.

Although Rorion was smart, you had to keep your eye on him, because he was a smooth talker. One day, when I was around eight, Rorion got home from school, and I asked him to take me to the beach. "Yes," he said, "but first," and took off his school belt and handed it to me, "this needs to be polished." Next, he took off his shoes and handed them to me. "And these need to be shined." I polished his brass belt buckle, shined his shoes, and then gave everything back to him.

"OK, I'm finished! Let's go to the beach."

"Not now! Get me some water and an apple. I'm hungry."

"Fuck, Rorion."

"No, go get me a fuckin' apple!"

I was pissed, but I got the apple and watched him eat it. "Can we go to the beach now?"

"No, not now."

"Fuck, Rorion, you've been exploiting me like a slave for hours. Fuck you!"

I ran to my room and slammed the door behind me. I learned at a young age to drive hard bargains with him.

Like Rolls, Rorion was one of the first Gracies to travel to the United States, and he introduced us to Jimi Hendrix and Santana. He told us stories about the music festivals he attended where people walked around naked and fucked in public like wild animals. We had hippie posters in our rooms, and it was a big deal when a new album came out. My dad and uncle tried to ignore our strange new habits and hairstyles, but they were impossible to ignore with my brother Relson in the mix.

Eight years older than me, Relson might have been the best fighter in the family if he wasn't such a wild man. Relson would show up at a tournament having had no sleep, still hungover from a night on the town. But when he put on his gi and tied his belt, he turned into a Tasmanian devil. Relson would fight all day, almost die . . . but win! Even though drugs were not supposed to be part of being a Gracie, most of us experimented with marijuana, cocaine, and hallucinogens. Relson went further than the rest of us. He'd stay up for days on cocaine. One time, he overdosed in our bathroom, and

Rolls saved his life. I remember once when he walked into the living room and I noticed that his shoulders were narrower than his hips. He looked like a walking skeleton. I realized that there were consequences to taking drugs.

I idolized all of my older brothers, but when I saw that Rolls and Rorion were worried about Relson's drug use, I got scared for him and became my dad's unofficial spy. I would go into his room, find his drugs, and give them to my dad. Even though it was obvious that Relson was going down the wrong road, Hélio let him and all of us make our own choices. He'd say to Relson, "If you go down this path, you're going to fuck yourself up! But you do whatever you are going to do." One day my dad said to me, "Relson is lost, but he has the heart to find the right path again. If he does, he'll be number one in the family!" My dad always pushed people to be their best, but didn't cut their heads off if they fell short. Hélio was a master, not a dictator, and he led with passion and love.

I was not interested in picking apart my brothers' flaws. Instead, I tried to take the things that I admired about them—emotional, technical, and strategic—and incorporate them into my own life. As I began to absorb and learn, I realized that I was in a position to be the greatest Gracie fighter of all time, because I had both the physical and the mental attributes. Rorion was also passionate about Jiu Jitsu but did not have my natural ability. Rolls was a great athlete, but he was stubborn and unmanageable. Relson was a natural warrior but lacked self-discipline.

My father could seem nice and light-hearted, but when he stepped onto the Jiu Jitsu mats, he was all business. Each weekend and on holidays, all of the Gracies would gather at our twenty-one-bedroom *casa grande* in Teresópolis. Thanks to the business acumen of Carlos's disciple George Santa Maria, my father and uncle were able to buy this house and the entire floor in the Rio office building where the academy was. Not only was the house huge, but there were gardeners, cooks, and seamstresses. Each weekend, my dad or my uncle drove all the dirty gis and towels from the academy to our ranch in Teresópolis, where the staff washed them in industrial washing machines, dried them on giant clotheslines, and folded them so they were ready to go back to Rio on Monday. It was a two-hour drive from Rio. Sometimes I would go there with Uncle Carlos in a pickup truck full of gis; other times my dad would drive me there in his Dodge Charger.

Once we got to Teresópolis, we rode horses and had big soccer games; friends came to visit, and there were luxuries like breakfast in bed. Every day, however, Hélio rolled a big canvas tarp out on the lawn, and all the boys had to train. We were his chicks that he was preparing to become roosters. My cousin Carlson was the reigning family champion, but he was seventeen years older than me, and the end of his fighting career was in sight. We all wondered who would be the next family champion, and the competition to see who would take his place was fierce.

Hélio encouraged competition among us and always

wanted to see who stood where in the Gracie food chain. There were confrontations and tests. My dad would step onto the canvas tarp, clap his hands, and say, "OK! Rolls–Rorion, go!" and without hesitation they would step forward to spar. Rolls and Rorion had totally different attitudes toward life, which were reflected in their Jiu Jitsu. There was never any question that Rolls was the best of our generation. Naturally, this was the hardest on Rorion. Not only did *he* want to be the family champion and the ambassador of Gracie Jiu Jitsu, but our dad also wanted him to be the champ, which added even more pressure.

In theory, Rorion was perfect! He had perfect technique, a perfect physique, and a perfect mind-set, but even with my dad barking instructions at him like a cornerman, Rolls whipped him every time. After he lost, dad could not mask his disappointment. He'd say, "Good job, Rolls," and then berate Rorion for his mistakes. It was sometimes hard to watch because they both gave everything they had. Rolls was just better. I think this is why Rorion gravitated to the business side of Jiu Jitsu.

My dad believed that suffering was part of the growth process, and we were programmed to believe that this theory was normal. We trained so hard in the academy that tournaments seemed easy. Hélio believed that the harder you trained, the easier you fought. We learned at a very young age that there was no point in chickening out, because it wouldn't get you out of anything. My dad would simply say, "Get back out there and do it again." You also realized that if you followed the Gracie protocols on training, diet, and fighting, they worked. Even my younger brother Royce, who is a very mellow guy, got pushed hard in training and understood commitment and suffering at a very young age.

There was always some drama in Teresópolis because we were all stretching ourselves to the limit. You either won or you lost, and all of your brothers and cousins saw it. Some rose to the challenge; others collapsed under the weight of it. My first Jiu Jitsu rival was a cousin who was a year older, but about my same size. Even though he was really competitive, I beat him regularly. One day he said to me, "You only beat me because we were wearing gis! Now you're not and I can beat you!" I smacked him, we started to fight, and I waited for him to get mad, because when he got mad, he bit his thumb, kept it in his mouth, and fought one-handed. This was his fatal flaw as a fighter. Sure enough, my cousin got mad and started biting his thumb, so I controlled him with one hand and punched him with other.

There were rivalries between Uncle Carlos's sons and Hélio's sons, but Rolls helped to mitigate these. Because he was Carlos's son who was raised by my dad and was the best fighter of our generation, Rolls brought the two sides of the family together. And since my brothers and I lived in Rio and were in the academy every day, we had an advantage over our cousins who grew up in Teresópolis. Some of my cousins thought Hélio was too harsh and training with him was too tough. My dad never tolerated excuses and often told people things that they did not want to hear about themselves. I think he treated his children and nephews the same. Rolls, after all, was really his nephew. He definitely favored his biological son, Rorion, but once it was undeniable that Rolls was the better fighter, Hélio offered no excuses and accepted the truth. If nothing else, my dad was a realist.

Our hierarchy was a brutally honest one, but we also learned to admit when we were wrong. If you told on your brother, Hélio would say, "I don't care who did what. If you both believe that you are right, I'll mediate a solution. But if one of you is lying, your punishment will be harsh because you knew what you did was wrong!" His approach ensured that we policed ourselves and realized it was best to solve our problems without getting dad involved.

When Hélio realized how good and how passionate I was about Jiu Jitsu, we developed a special relationship. My dad recognized something in me and encouraged me to become the greatest Gracie. He never had to push me the way he had to push some of the others.

In addition to Jiu Jitsu, my father and I also shared a great passion for animals. He and Uncle Carlos treated animals like people. They did not try to tame them as much as they made friends with them. My uncle liked to sunbathe naked on top of the water tower, and he befriended two wild hawks in Teresópolis. My dad liked to adopt the meanest dogs he could find, the ones that bit everyone, and then turn them into his pets. It was yet another test for him.

I don't know if it was patience or mind control, but nobody was better with dogs than my father. He believed that

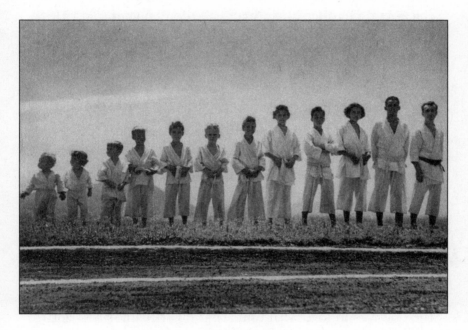

SOME OF CARLOS AND HÉLIO GRACIE'S SONS.
PHOTOGRAPH COURTESY OF THE RICKSON GRACIE COLLECTION.

the strength of his mind allowed him to connect with even the most vicious animals of any species. His friend owned a crazy Doberman that bit everyone, so my dad started going by his house just to visit the dog. They got so close that when Hélio left, the Doberman would cry until my dad came back the next time to see him. Finally, the dog's owner said, "Hélio, I'm giving you the dog, because the only time he's happy is when you're around." Soon, my dad had a kennel full of Doberman pinschers.

João, another one of my dad's friends, bred filas (mastiffs). These gigantic, aggressive dogs weigh over a hundred pounds and were once used to hunt big game and runaway slaves in Brazil. He had one really mean dog, called Booma, who at the age of six months attacked João, so he gave him to my dad. João put a leash on the dog, and he, my dad, and Booma drove up to our ranch. When they arrived, Hélio took him out of the car by the leash and did not let go of that leash for the whole weekend. My dad finally took Booma off it and the dog was in love with him. That dog became good with kids and was loved by the whole family. Next, he got a German shepherd named Thor, who became my first dog.

Hélio also liked horses and mules, especially the ones that kicked apart their corrals, the ones that the toughest Brazilian cowboys thought were crazy. When I was ten, my dad gave me a mare I named Lauren, who was my first love. In the late 1960s, my father bought a fifty-acre ranch of his own in a beautiful valley in Petropolis. He called it Nosso Vale (Our Valley). I spent my days there cleaning and grooming Lauren. I was the first person to mount her and was eventually able to ride her bareback without a bridle. Using only my legs, I could command her to speed up, slow down, stop, turn right, left. There was a real synchronicity between us. I'd feed her carrots, and she would kiss me and follow me around without a lead rope. If I put a child on her back, she knew to be gentle.

My dad's horse, Mustang, was a Paso Fino stallion that looked like Roy Rogers's horse, Trigger. He lived in a grassy field with Lauren and the other mares. One day, my dad told me to bring Mustang down from the top of the pasture. I put a lead rope around his neck and started to bring him down the hill, but he began to drag me, so I stopped and mounted him. Mustang saw that someone had left the corral open. He ran right onto the dirt road and began to gallop toward the highway. My dad saw the disaster that was unfolding and screamed, "Hold on!" just before we vanished over the hill.

I grabbed the stallion's mane as he galloped downhill. Mustang was not stupid. As he got closer to the highway, he slowed down enough for me to jump off. I landed on my feet, grabbed the lead rope, regained control of the horse, and calmed him. Then I remounted him and started to ride back to the ranch. Just as we crested the hill, I saw my dad running toward us. When he saw me and Mustang calmly riding back to the ranch, he screamed, "Yes!" and the fear in his eyes turned to pride. The connection we made that day was a real victory for me because I had proved to Hélio that his confidence in me was not misplaced, and my dad was never scared for me again. If anything, he was over-confident in me and gave me a great deal of freedom that I made the most of.

I was by myself a lot because I was so much younger than my brothers. I never needed people around me to feel comfortable, and I was extremely curious about the world. When I rode my bike through Copacabana, Thor would run next to me. If I rode in the street, he would follow me on the sidewalk. If I crossed a street, he'd wait on the curb until I said, "Go!" and then he'd sprint through traffic jams and busy streets. It didn't matter to him. If I went somewhere in a car with my friends, I'd leave my bike on the sidewalk and say, "Sit right here!" Thor would wait for hours.

Rio is like New York City and Bangkok combined. It is a turbulent, whatever-you-want-whenever-you-want-it mix of sex, crime, drugs, nature, and beach culture. Although we lived in a nice apartment in Copacabana, Rio is not like LA. There is not a rich town like Beverly Hills and then a poor one like Compton; they are combined. One minute you're in Beverly Hills and the next you turn down a side street and are in Compton. As a kid, I developed street smarts. At every stoplight there is a group of guys who are that block's eyes and ears. Some sell drinks, some sell candy, and some sell drugs. If a car stops, they approach the driver's window and if the driver just stares ahead like they don't exist, he might get a rock through the window, and lose his wallet.

From the gangbangers, to the fighters, to the high-society matrons, to the surfers, to the most beautiful girls in

Ipanema, I wanted to understand all of it. I would often ditch school and just walk around Rio. I had normal rounds that I made through the city.

First I would visit the appliance store and joke around with the salesman. "You want to buy a refrigerator, kid?" he'd ask.

"Not today, but maybe tomorrow!"

Then I would go to the bakery, buy a snack, and talk with the baker. Next, it was off to the newsstand to talk to the guy who sold papers about the recent soccer matches. Everyone knew that I was supposed to be in school because I was still wearing my uniform and carrying my books; I guess I provided some relief from their daily grinds.

Many of the upper-class kids seemed dumb to me because they had no street smarts. I didn't want to be a sheltered kid who knew nothing about real life and lived inside of a comfortable bubble. Sometimes my mom's rich friends would come over to our house with their sons who were around my age, and it was difficult for me to relate to them because I grew up with much older brothers. They'd want to talk about the new Walt Disney movie, and I'd want to talk about the latest issue of *Playboy* or the new Led Zeppelin album. After they left, my mom would ask, "Did you like little José?"

"He was a spoiled little shit!"

"Why don't you like him?"

"He's not smart, Mom! He doesn't know anything about anything!"

I was beginning to understand that money and social position defined some people, but I wanted to be defined by my merit. Brazil's population comes from all over the world. There are European Brazilians, African Brazilians, Japanese Brazilians, Indian African Brazilians, and just about any other racial and ethnic combination you can imagine.

Class, on the other hand, was a different matter, because the rich didn't mix with the poor. My grandfather was a wealthy man who owned a department store and a great deal of real estate. My mother, Margarida, was very well traveled, spoke French, and was a member of Rio's high society. Her father was not happy when she fell madly in love with "a fighter" whom he considered beneath his daughter's social status.

I learned about class the hard way. One day when I was seven or eight, I went down to the beach by myself and started playing with a kid from the favela who was also alone. We were digging tunnels in the sand and having a lot of fun together. A couple of hours later, I brought the boy back to our apartment for lunch. When we walked in, my mother looked at the kid and asked, "Why'd you bring him here?"

"He's my friend, Mom! We came to eat, and then we're going back to the beach to play some more."

My mother made us lunch, but I felt that I had done something wrong. I was surprised by both my mom's fearful reaction and the fact that she doubted my judgment.

It was very uncomfortable, so when I came home later, I asked her what was wrong, and she said, "That boy is so poor, you shouldn't play with him! He might come here one day and steal your things." This particular kid was smart, courageous, tough, someone I felt very aligned with. I thought to myself, *My mother is trying to forbid me from being friends with him just because he is poor!* The message that I took away from that experience was probably the opposite of the one that my mother was trying to send. I disagreed strongly with the idea that I should judge people by their appearance or social status. Instead, I decided to follow my heart. Money can't buy the most important things in life. Friendship, loyalty, courage, honesty, happiness, intelligence—anyone from any class, race, or station in life may or may not have these attributes. If I felt power, love, respect, intelligence, I was going to engage with an open heart and be willing to accept that person as a brother or sister.

If anything, my mom's attitude made the streets seem even more attractive. The kids were smarter, they didn't get ripped off, and they knew how to take care of themselves because they were more experienced. At thirteen, I decided to stop going to school because it seemed pointless to me. I loved Jiu Jitsu and surfing and knew that I was going to be a fighter. What did I need school for? I told my dad that I was dropping out of school and he wisely said, "You are still my son. I will feed you, but don't bother me for anything else. No new bicycles or presents—from now on you have to make your own money."

The first cash I ever made was from helping Rorion teach

Jiu Jitsu. Soon I found more-lucrative hustles than working for my brother. While I am not proud of my flirtation with the criminal lifestyle, I think it is important that I acknowledge it. My experiences on the streets of Rio were priceless and helped to shape me; they allowed me to taste forbidden fruits and to enter worlds I never would have otherwise. Today I try to lead by example, and do not advocate using illegal drugs or many legal ones. There are too many people searching for pharmaceutical solutions to basic human problems. Temporary depression is a natural human reaction to the loss of a loved one or other misfortunes in life. How can a pill change something like that? Today, if a child has trouble concentrating in school, his parents don't take away his iPhone, iPad, and computer and make him play outside. Instead, they go to a psychiatrist, who prescribes medication for his condition. Illegal drugs like black-market Fentanyl, as well as prescription opiates, are so powerful and addictive that to take them is to gamble with your life. While I am not proud to expose this part of my history, I have to be honest. If I hadn't had these experiences, I would be a very different person.

I made myself examine and try to understand everything I was curious about. I sought out new and extreme experiences. I knew that I could get hurt, but I decided the risk was worth it. I know many excellent Jiu Jitsu fighters whose minds are not open because they are scared and threatened by ideas and lifestyles they do not understand. The first thing they do is judge, often without any basis. I try not to be judgmental but to accept things as they are, not how I would like them to be. Even though I had helped my father try to pull Relson from the hole of drug addiction, part of me also wanted to see what lurked inside that hole.

I was fourteen when I fell in with a gang of teenagers who lived in an apartment complex where my uncle Carlos had an apartment. We called ourselves Camões, after the housing project where most of them lived. There were thirty or forty of us, between the ages of fourteen and twenty. We were an army of streetwise kids who were trying to capitalize on anything and everything we could. We didn't care if you were rich or poor; if you were in sync with us mentally, physically, and emotionally, you were our brother. The only way that you could become part of our group was by your individual merit.

Some of the smartest, most courageous people I've ever met were in that gang. I knew they would back me—win or lose, right or wrong—no matter what. Given that toughness, loyalty, and courage were the values my family held sacred, I wanted to be around people who shared those values. Initially, I was one of the youngest kids, but the older guys liked me because I made myself useful. There was a handful of rich guys in our gang, but the majority were middle- and lower-class. If you said, "Let's go to the restaurant and eat filet mignon," only one guy would go with you, but if you said, "Let's go rob the popcorn stand," everyone would go.

Camões had a beach soccer team. *Beasal*, or beach soccer, was invented in Rio during the 1950s. It's just like regular soccer except that there are only five players per side and the field is just forty yards long. When I was growing up, there were five or six teams that represented different Copacabana neighborhoods. The competition was fierce, and hundreds of people would turn out for the big tournaments. The Camões guys used to like to stand behind our rival's goal and try to distract their goalie by yelling insults at him. There was always tension at those games, and afterward it would usually explode with a few fights and lots of chaos and commotion. One time we went to Urca, where Camões was playing. After a referee's disputed call, one of the leaders of Camões started fighting with a fan from the rival team. Very quickly we were outnumbered, almost surrounded, and had to run for our lives back to Copacabana with a hundred of the other team's supporters on our heels. We would stop and fight a little bit and then keep running. These fights were not personal; it was more like team against team. Somebody might occasionally throw a bottle, but there were never any guns like today.

Very quickly, I proved myself brave and reliable and began to move up the Camões food chain. First, I worked as a lookout and messenger for a pot dealer named Clayo. When it got dark, he would go down to the beach and stand near the ocean because there he could see everyone, but nobody could see him. Next, I started making deliveries and selling pot myself. Because I lived a half hour away in a more upper-middle-class area, I became the airplane that dropped weed into my neighborhood.

One day a friend wanted to buy a small bag. I was in a

rush, so I took a handful of pot out of a much bigger one-pound bag. Instead of putting the pound bag in its hiding place, I put it under the pillow on my bed and ran out of the house. When I got home, the bag of weed was gone and I knew I was in deep shit. I was more afraid of Clayo than my mom, so I asked her for my pot back. "I don't want to talk to you! I'm going to show it to your dad," she said. Then Rorion came home, and he tried to interrogate me, but I refused to talk to anyone but my dad. When Hélio finally got home, he and Rorion started flushing the pot down the toilet. I begged them not to do it because the weed was not mine! The second the words left my lips, I knew I had made a mistake. Now all eyes were on me. My dad now wanted to know who was fronting a pound of pot to a fourteen-year-old. Worse, Hélio wanted me to take him to talk to Clayo the next night! "I'm not going to arrest him or beat him up," my dad promised. "I'm just going to tell him to stay away from you."

The next night, we went to the beach, and I approached Clayo with my dad and Rorion. "Clayo, my dad wants to . . ."

Hélio cut me off. "Hey motherfucker! If you ever . . ." The dealer tried to run for it, but Rorion tackled him and held him down as my dad lectured him menacingly. He begged for forgiveness and was totally humiliated. The next morning, I felt horrible, so I went to see Clayo. I offered to work off the pot and promised that it would never happen again. He forgave me. Even though I went back into business for a little while longer, I began to drift away from

Camões when members started stealing stereos and using guns. I knew they were on a path that would take them nowhere fast, and I was much more interested in Jiu Jitsu, surfing, and girls than a life of crime. Although I was rebellious and did things that my dad didn't agree with, I never stopped competing and never stopped winning. In his eyes, this made me special.

It was about this time that I began to train with my brother Rolls. Up to this point, Hélio was my only teacher. Whether he was surfing, training, fighting, riding horses, hang gliding, or chasing girls, Rolls was constantly in motion. He was fast, technical, and always pushed me to train harder and achieve more. Initially, he was teaching with my father and Rorion downtown. Then Rolls started teaching three days a week at my cousin Carlson's school in Copacabana. After he retired as family champion, Carlson was the first member of the second generation of Gracies to break with my father. He opened his own school in 1964 and, unlike Hélio, taught group classes and even allowed students to train for free as long as they were good fighters and willing to carry the Gracie flag into battle. Carlson's generosity is legendary, which explains the loyalty and gratitude that so many fighters have for him even today.

My cousin's academy was the opposite of my father's. It was filthy! Everyone wore dirty gis and when you walked in you got intimidated by the smell alone! Carlson's students were aggressive, but relied too much on strength. His techniques weren't the most polished, but they fit with the kind of students he had. My cousin's teaching style was also brutal. When my dad was coaching a student, he would say, "OK, stay calm, maintain your base, and work your escape." In the same situation, Carlson would have screamed at the student, "Get your fucking head out of there and smash that motherfucker!" To him, Gracie Jiu Jitsu wasn't about the triumph of brains over brawn or precise technique or the family diet; it was all about fighting until your heart came out of your mouth. If you could survive training in that environment, tournaments were just another day at the office.

I started to go to Carlson's academy in Copacabana to train because there were more students my age. The downtown academy was mostly businessmen taking private lessons, and therefore the training was much softer. My cousin's school was the opposite. It was packed with tough young guys who wanted to become fighters. It was a much more intense and dynamic environment. You never knew who might show up to train with Rolls because he was also training in Judo, Sambo, and wrestling.

Rolls wanted to establish a Brazilian national wrestling team to compete internationally. This irritated the officials of Brazil's official wrestling governing body, who considered us upstarts who were trying to encroach on their turf. In 1978, FILA (Fédération Internationale des Luttes Associées, or International Federation of Associated Wrestling Styles, now named United World Wrestling), the world's governing body for wrestling, sent American wrestler Bob Anderson to Rio to coach the Brazilian wrestlers who were Rolls's rivals.

Anderson was a big and extremely skilled Greco-Roman, Freestyle, and Sambo champion from Southern California who was also a good surfer.

When Bob Anderson arrived in Rio, nobody from the official wrestling organization came to pick him up at the airport. Someone who knew Rolls saw the giant, muscular American who looked like the Incredible Hulk waiting with his surfboard at the airport and struck up a conversation with him. Somehow, word reached Rolls that an American wrestling champion was stranded at the airport. By the time he and my cousin Carlson showed up at the airport, Anderson had been waiting for hours.

According to legend, Rolls apologized for being late, told Anderson they were the "Brazilian wrestling officials," put his board on the roof of the car, and off they went. For the next week, Anderson and Rolls lived, trained, and surfed together; Bob even got to go to a Brazil-versus-Argentina soccer game. Rio with Rolls was another level of fun and constant activity.

By the time the American wrestler realized that he had been kidnapped by my brother, he didn't want to leave. But it wasn't all fun and games. Anderson and Rolls trained hard and compared and dissected each other's techniques. The wrestler thought it was strange that Rolls always wore a gi, but he was having so much fun that he didn't ask too many questions. What impressed the American most was Rolls's ability to work out of any position. He would later call Rolls "a renaissance man" who took elements from other martial arts, even other sports, and applied them to Jiu Jitsu.

Bob Anderson helped Rolls modify a wrestling hold called a keylock, which Rolls renamed the Americana in his honor. Today, it is a popular Jiu Jitsu submission. Just before Anderson left to go home, he and Rolls had a match. They went back and forth for a long time before Rolls caught him in a heel hook. Bob Anderson was a gracious guest who really connected with Rolls and the Gracie family.

Training with Rolls was essentially fighting. He reinforced what Hélio had already taught me: *Fuck points! Fuck judges! Win by submission or not at all.* I began to improve quickly under Rolls, and Hélio was not surprised. I wasn't stubborn and never choked under pressure. Now the expectations for me were from both Rolls and my dad, and they were extremely high.

My dad was never euphoric after my victories; he expected me to win. Now he needed me, because I was always ready to fight challengers to prove that his Jiu Jitsu was the best. Hélio loved to take me to my cousin Carlson's academy. "You think your Jiu Jitsu is better than mine?" he'd say to Carlson. "My kid can beat your best guys!"

Carlson Gracie was a warm-hearted guy, but he was also super competitive. It didn't matter if it was a cockfight, a poker game, or a *vale tudo* match; he was most comfortable in the center of turmoil and chaos. He used to piss everyone off at tournaments because he would scream at the referees and totally intimidate them. The biggest rivalry at that time was between Carlson and Rolls. At tournaments, we could have only two athletes fight in each belt and weight division.

The qualifying tournaments between Rolls's students, Carlson's students, and Rorion's students to see who was going to represent us were always more competitive than the actual tournaments. Eventually, we separated the schools. Rolls and Rorion's students would represent the Gracie Academy and Carlson's students would represent the Carlson Gracie Academy.

By the time father awarded me my purple belt at sixteen, I was getting good at spotting my opponents' flaws and capitalizing on them. I had many tough matches, but I always won, and was really starting to feel my power. One day, a friend and student took me to the Luta Livre academy at Boqueirão for some no-gi training. There were about twenty guys there, and they had no idea who I was. My friend just told the teacher, "I brought a friend to spar with us. He has a background in Jiu Jitsu." The teacher said, "No problem," pointed to one of the biggest guys in the room, and said to me, "Spar with him." After I beat the big guy easily, he said, "Now, spar with him," and pointed to another big guy. In less than an hour, I had submitted everyone in the class but the teacher. We had a match, and after I submitted him, it was a bit awkward until my friend said, "You've got nothing to be ashamed of. That's Hélio Gracie's son Rickson."

"Well fuck! That explains it," the teacher said. "I have a lot of respect for your dad. Come back anytime."

While I liked grappling and Jiu Jitsu competitions, I was already thinking about my first *vale tudo* fight. Today, it is possible to get a Jiu Jitsu black belt without knowing self-defense or even getting into a real fight. This was impossible during the 1970s and 1980s. Because my father and uncle loudly proclaimed their style "the world's most effective form of self-defense," every young Gracie knew that at some point he would be called upon to represent our family in the ring or in the street. Your first official *vale tudo* fight was like losing your virginity; it was a rite of passage.

PREDATORS AND PREY

AS I BEGAN TO UNDERSTAND HOW TRANSFORMATIVE JIU JITSU was, I fell in love with teaching and my ability to change people and their behavior from within. It was much more than teaching Jiu Jitsu; it was also adding something to someone's life. My father taught me that if you want to be a great instructor, you need to think of Jiu Jitsu not only as techniques to be taught, but as a psychological education as well. In addition to fighting, students learn how to better sense danger, the difference between patience and passivity, and how losing is not the same thing as being defeated. First you have to understand your students as people. If they're too excitable, mellow them out. If they're too mellow, light a fire under their ass. If they're passive, make them more aggressive. My dad and Rorion taught me how to teach the entire person—including the psyche—and not just the fighter.

When I put physical pressure on students, I see their true personalities because they immediately show me things that they are able to hide when they're not on the mat: their state of emotional balance or ability to manage pressure, for example. Once I have this information, I use it to tailor a curriculum to the students' needs that will benefit each of them in a profound way. I don't make them examine just how they fight, but also how they *feel* when they fight. If students do this honestly, they don't just get better at Jiu Jitsu; they rebuild themselves as stronger people. They learn how to be tougher, smarter, more resilient—not just in a fight, but also in everyday life.

I was around seventeen when I met Sergio Zveiter at the academy downtown and began to teach him privately. He was twenty or twenty-one and had just graduated from law school, but I knew even then that he would go far in law or maybe politics. We became good friends and would often go out to eat after class and surf together. Because we were both very accomplished in our own fields, we had a great deal of mutual respect that grew into a deep bond, and Sergio later became my most trusted adviser. It was not just his sharp mind that I liked; he was also a very straight shooter. If I had a question, I would always ask him what he thought,

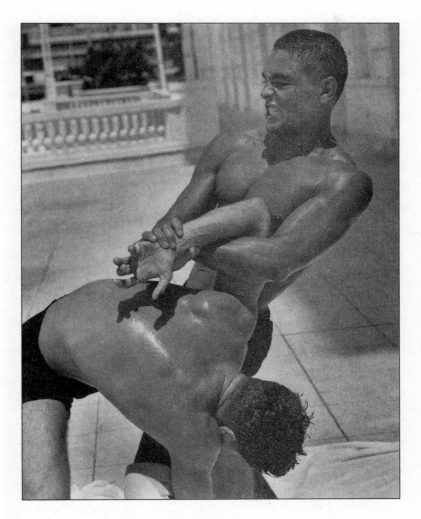

RICKSON GRACIE, RIO.
PHOTOGRAPH COURTESY OF BRUCE WEBER.

because I knew that he would always give me his honest opinion whether I liked it or not.

By seventeen, I was a full Jiu Jitsu instructor and made more money than a bank manager. If I was not training, I was spending my time at the beach in Ipanema with the surfers. Unlike my gangster friends, who were much more intense and interested only in fucking and fighting, the surfers were hippies and lovers. Our lives were centered on the waves and beach. The sea has always been a great normalizer for me. If I'm tense and I go into the ocean, I come out relaxed. If I'm lazy and tired and I go in, I come away energized. The ocean either gives me the extra energy that I need or takes away the excess energy that I don't. Rivers and waterfalls do similar things for me. When I was a kid, I liked to stay in the ocean until I was freezing cold, then go on the beach and roll in the hot sand to warm up. First I rode inflatable surf mats, then Styrofoam boards, and eventually moved up to real surfboards.

I realized that the sea was a place where I could test myself and push my limits. The ocean is too strong to fight; you have to flow with it, remain calm, and navigate your way in and out of incredibly complex situations. One day around this time, I was at the beach checking the surf on a stormy day. Nobody was around because it was windy and out of control. Then I noticed a skinny kid with long hair at the water's edge with a red surfboard. It turned out that it was my brother Rolls's friend Pepe, who was one of Brazil's first big-wave riders. I sat down and watched him paddle out into the violent sea and then surf with a kind of casual grace and mastery that I had never seen before. Pepe was a little older than me but not by much. If he could surf like this, then so could I. I was now on a mission to get my black belt in surfing.

Surfing was a new sport in Brazil, so it was a big deal when the first professional surfing contest came to Rio in 1977. My brothers and I all surfed and were excited to see our Hawaiian, Australian, and Californian idols. My friend Foca was surfing our local beach, and he collided with a Hawaiian pro surfer named Byron Amona, who was a member of the infamous Hawaiian surf gang the Black Shorts. They ruled Oahu's North Shore and were nasty to outsiders, especially Brazilians. The big Hawaiian grabbed Foca's board, punched the fins out, and kicked him out of the water at his home beach! Can you imagine the humiliation?

I was at Ipanema Beach right after it happened, and Foca showed up with his broken board and told us that the big Hawaiian had punched out his fins and kicked him out of the water. We went to find Amona, but he had already left. That night, I told my dad and brothers what had happened at the beach, and everyone agreed that Amona needed to be put in his place. The Hawaiian needed to know that the rules were different here in Brazil.

A day or so later, we found out that Byron Amona and some other Hawaiian and American pro surfers were at the home and surfboard factory of Brazil's first pro surfer, Rico de Souza. Everyone in Rio knew that the Gracies drove

Volkswagens, so when the Brazilian surfboard factory workers saw a fleet of VWs pull up and us pile out, they ran for their lives. One guy even jumped out of a window. My brother Relson came, but most of the other twenty with us were surfers.

Everyone waited outside while I went inside Rico's factory to find Byron Amona. When I saw Byron's Dick Brewer surfboard, I told a friend to grab it and take it outside. I found Rico in his shaping room talking with one of the Americans, and I told him that we had a problem that needed to be resolved. "This motherfucker Byron broke Foca's board and now needs to pay for it one way or another." Once Rico sensed that I was in fighting mode, he said, "Please, let's go outside," and tried to usher us out of the house. When Rico saw the crowd outside, he knew where this was going and said, "Please, Rickson, don't destroy my business!" I told Rico that if he wanted to kiss the Hawaiians' asses and let them act like assholes in his own hometown, he could fight too! Rico tried to deescalate the situation, but he was stuck between a rock and a hard place.

As I was walking back outside, I peeked into the side yard and saw pro surfers Mike Purpus, Michael Ho, and Byron Amona smoking a joint. They looked at me, laughed, and flashed me shaka hand signs with their fingers. I didn't smile back and stared at Amona instead. Thirty seconds later, the Hawaiian was outside screaming, "Where's my board? Where's my board?"

Everyone got quiet, and then I said in Portuguese, "Your board is with me."

He looked at me with contempt. There was more silence, which I broke with the only English phrases I knew: "Fuck you, motherfucker! I'm going to break your face!" The Hawaiian didn't take me seriously because I was a 150-pound eighteen-year-old and he was over 250 pounds.

Byron realized that I had just challenged him to fight, and he began to loosen up his arms and legs like a kickboxer. He turned to Rico and said, "I'm going to hurt this kid." I shot in, got him in a clinch, tripped him, and took him down. Amona tried to stand up, but I took his back, choked him out, and he fell on his face unconscious. I punched him back to his senses, and when he tried to stand up again, I got his back and started to choke him out for the second time. Amona was really strong, so I couldn't finish the choke and head-butted him instead. "Put this motherfucker to sleep!" Relson yelled as Rico begged, "Please don't kill him!" After I put Byron to sleep for the second time, I grabbed a piece of concrete and smashed his board with it. It only seemed fair, given what he had done to Foca.

Word of the fight spread quickly. The next day, some of the Australian pro surfers came up to me at the beach and said, "Fuck! You're the guy who beat Byron. I wish I knew your techniques!" They congratulated me and were happy because the Black Shorts gang and Amona made their lives miserable in Hawaii. A few days later, I saw Byron Amona at the opening ceremony of the Waimea 5000 surf contest drinking beer with his friends. He started yelling and got very aggressive. His friends held him back as he screamed,

"I'm going to find you and kick your ass!" After that, Amona started telling people that he was going to find me and "get me" before he returned to Hawaii. When I told my dad about these threats, he said that we would pay the Hawaiian a visit at his hotel. The next day, my dad, Rorion, and I went to the Sheraton Hotel at Leblon. The hotel has its own private beach, so I waited there while Rorion, the only one of us who spoke English, went inside. He found Byron by the swimming pool, introduced himself, and told him that I was waiting for him on the beach. "You either fight Rickson now or forget the matter," Rorion explained. "You said that you were going to 'find him,' and that is not acceptable." Byron told my brother that he didn't want to fight again and that the matter was resolved. The Hawaiian went home a few days later with a better understanding of Brazil. I'd like to think we were his unofficial cultural ambassadors.

Such an easy win against such an intimidating guy gave me a great deal of confidence, perhaps even overconfidence. After that fight, the best surfers in Rio began to show me respect, and even the girls took notice. I was often frustrated in Ipanema because the beautiful beach girls my age usually dated rich guys with convertibles. That would soon change.

It was around this time that I began to realize that my father and uncle were frozen in time. Everything from their relationships with the women in their lives to their views on procreation seemed out of touch. How the fuck was I supposed to have sex only for procreation and never masturbate? You have to realize that sex in Brazil is much freer and more natural than in the United States. The weather is hot and humid, people wear very few clothes, and we are impulsive, sensual people who like to be in close contact to each other. The sweat, the physical intimacy, the sensations—Brazilians need this proximity and bodily engagement to feel comfortable. For many Brazilians, sex is like eating; it is just a human need. My father and uncles had a different view of this—as evidenced by their legacy of children—but I wanted the enjoyable aspects of sex as well. I wanted the passion and fun.

Drugs were plentiful in Rio when I was growing up. No matter what experiences I had with drugs, I always felt that I had a strong base. I was loved and protected at home, which left me free to dream, venture out into the world, and find my place in it. If my dad had said, "Don't do that! That is wrong!" my story would be a very different one. As Gracies, we were all taught the protocols on fighting, diet, and training, but it was our decision to follow them or not. The lack of pressure, ironically, made me feel more grounded.

Surfers liked marijuana and hallucinogens like magic mushrooms. We used to go to the cow pastures to pick the golden mushrooms that grew in the cow shit. We would eat the foul-tasting fungus with lime and then go to the beach, paddle out into the surf, and wait for the trip to start. I remember one day when the waves were small but perfect. As the mushrooms came on, I felt like I could see the atoms in the water. Then I felt like an amphibious creature who could stay underwater for as long as I wanted. After I got out of the sea, I walked to a rocky area and my feet felt like part of the rock. I stayed planted there for hours. This experience forced me to look outside of myself and to marvel at the beauty of the natural world.

By the time I was seventeen, Rio's night life was playing a bigger role in my life. Typically, a night out would consist of visiting different nightclubs and not getting home until after sunrise. Sometimes we would just walk around and listen for music. If we heard a party, we'd figure out which apartment it was in and crash it. We drank whisky like the cowboys in movies, and Rio, so close to Peru, was awash in pure cocaine. Because I was not exactly square, I certainly tried it, but my family support system made it hard to go too far astray because I knew that the next day, tired or not, I would be teaching and training.

Some of my friends who didn't have this type of support had begun to slip. One night I would see them at the club, and a month later I'd see them staggering around the street barefoot. "Fuck, man! What happened to your front teeth? Where's your motorcycle?" I'd ask.

"I don't know man. The last thing I remember is the night we were doing lines with those beautiful girls at the club!"

Sometimes after a big night out I'd feel I'd gone too far, but come the next day, I would eat well, run, surf, and train. I'd be good for a week or two, and then a voice in my head would direct me off path: "The night! The girls! They're waiting for you!" Even though drugs were more dangerous for my friends who were not athletes, I would learn that drug addiction can strike anyone.

Five years younger than me, Marcelo Behring was one of my best friends and best students. He was born into Jiu Jitsu royalty; his father, Flavio, was my dad's student and also an instructor. Marcelo grew up on the mat, and when he was fourteen, he started coming to my school to train with me. We immediately connected, and over time he became like another younger brother. Because Marcelo had been training since he was a little kid, I refined and built upon his existing knowledge. As he started to perfect his connections and other invisible aspects of Jiu Jitsu, he went from a good blue belt to one of my best students. Marcelo always competed under my flag, and I was always in his corner, pushing him to get better and better. As a brown belt, he fought and won an important *vale tudo* match and gained a great deal of respect. When I was in his corner, he could do anything.

When Marcelo was training with me in Brazil, he partied occasionally, maybe 5 percent of the time, but his main priority was training and fighting. After I left Brazil to pursue my own fighting career, he lost his direction and began partying 25 percent of the time. After he signed a contract for a professional fight and didn't show up, I think he felt ashamed and his downward spiral began. Every time we spoke, I tried to draw Marcelo toward the light and get him back to fighting and training. His family even put him in rehab, but he left early and could not break the grip of his cocaine addiction. I got really worried about him when one of our mutual friends told me that they had seen him walking around Rio at four a.m. in swim trunks. Shortly thereafter, he vanished, and his family didn't hear from him for three months. The Behrings hired a private investigator, who eventually found Marcelo's body in a pauper's grave. It was suspected that he was killed in a favela in a drug deal gone wrong. For some, the grip of addiction is too strong to break.

If I were to be the greatest Gracie, I had to take risks. Even though I experimented with different drugs and potentially dangerous lifestyles, I valued my freedom above all. I never wanted to be controlled by anything, especially a drug. I also realized that I had a God-given talent for Jiu Jitsu, and with this came the honor and responsibility to represent my family. This always brought me back to a place of equilibrium. It was always fun to leave reality for a night, but no matter what, I was back in the academy training the next day. I never knew who might walk through the door and challenge me, and becoming the greatest Gracie was more important to me than anything else.

Curiosity coupled with courage allows you to go beyond your limits, venture into the unknown, and establish new limits that you never thought were possible. My curiosity always overpowered my fear, but fear was also a good friend to me. People who say they are not afraid of anything are either crazy or stupid. Fear is a normal emotion that protects you, but sometimes you don't need protection. There are times when you have to place fear on the shelf and take action without a moment's hesitation. One such time occurred one evening when I was out alone surfing Saquarema, one of Brazil's best big wave breaks.

The sun was starting to set, but I decided to catch one more wave. As I was paddling back out, a clean-up set broke on my head, my leash broke, and I never saw my surfboard again. The current started to pull me out to sea. When I realized that it was too strong to swim against, a jolt of adrenaline snapped me to my senses. I knew that if I panicked or made a mistake, I would die. In order to get out of the current, I had to swim parallel to shore at a pace that would allow me to swim for hours, if necessary. I used the lights from a church way down the coast as a visual bearing and focused on my stroke and my breathing. Two hours later, when I stumbled onto dry land, I wasn't just happy to get back in. I was proud of myself because I had used my brain and my endurance to save my own life. Winning fights, riding wild horses, or taming vicious dogs—none of it compared to this. That swim was by far the most terrifying experience of my life, because nature was working against me. Luck did not get me back to shore: I faced down primal fear and prevailed. The next day, I made myself go back to Saquarema, paddle out, and catch a few waves.

I eventually learned that the capacity to accept anything, especially death, was the key to my physical, mental, and spiritual growth. All three of these elements must be balanced, because sometimes you don't break physically but emotionally. Sometimes you have the physicality and the emotional control but are spiritually unprepared. Without a spiritual connection to both life and death, you can't reach the next level of performance. Soon I would realize that if I were to dance on the razor's edge, I might fall off it and die. That was the price of admission.

By the time I was a brown belt, my matches with my brother Rolls were getting closer. I was beginning to understand the limitations of his game. Rolls had an excellent knee-on-belly move that he used to set up armlocks, and he was lethal if he got your back, but he was also predictably aggressive. In our final ten training sessions, not only did Rolls not submit me, but I was getting reversals, and our fights were now even.

One afternoon we were training together by ourselves at my dad's ranch in Petropolis. The only thing I remember is engaging with Rolls, then going through the eye of a hurricane with all the violence you would expect. When the storm passed, I had Rolls in a choke, and before I even realized what was happening, he was tapping. It was a completely reactive fight. I'm not even sure if I was mounted or on his back. All I remember is that I finished him with a choke. Nobody else saw me beat Rolls, and when we finished training, we hugged and he kissed me on the cheek and said, "You did good, kid. I'm proud of you."

What I remember most about that fight was the sadness I felt afterward, as though I had made a mistake by beating him. A huge but invisible weight of responsibility had shifted from Rolls's shoulders to mine. In my heart, I knew that I was now a better fighter, but worse, so did he. It wasn't luck or a fluke; Rolls just couldn't surprise me anymore. I also realized that I would never have to beat him again to prove it.

But things were different in public. When Rolls and I faced each other in open division finals of tournaments and the referee signaled the start of the match, I would walk across the mat and raise his hand in the air. Rolls would always take first, and I would take second. He and I knew that I was the best, but to the rest of the universe, Rolls was still the champion. I didn't need to announce to the world that I had defeated my brother. I didn't want to break his spirit and put myself above him. Keeping this secret was a way for me to honor him and my family.

By the time I got my black belt a few months after beating Rolls, he and I were going in completely different directions. My brother was putting all of his energy into competitive grappling in an effort to establish a Brazilian national wrestling team. American wrestler Bob Anderson, who had stayed with him in Rio, helped him navigate the international bureaucracy and got us invited to the 1979 world Sambo championships in San Diego. Invented in Russia, Sambo is a competitive grappling style that includes knee, ankle, and leg attacks. However, many of my favorite Jiu Jitsu submissions are not allowed. My dad paid for me, Rolls, and Carlos Jr. to go to America to compete in three different weight divisions.

When the competition began, we started to submit everyone with foot locks. The referees got mad because we were going only for submissions, not throws or points, so they began to stop our fights before we could submit our opponents. Once, Rolls caught one guy in a foot lock, and the referee stopped the match and said, "You can't grab the joint, only the shin!" Every time Rolls got near a foot, they stopped the match, so he ended up getting only third in his division. Carlos Jr. made the finals and lost. I made the finals and faced a strong wrestler from the US Air Force. He got on top of me and I couldn't sweep him because his base was excellent. He was up 15–0 with only one minute left when I finally swept him and mounted. He tried to push me off and I arm-locked him. He screamed in pain and the referee stopped the fight: I won my division. Even though I won the gold medal, I thought the tournament was bullshit. I was only allowed to use straight arm bars, foot locks, and knee bars, and even those were subject to a bunch of rules and subjective referee decisions.

Wrestling was even worse than Sambo when it came to arbitrary rules and biased referees. Rolls, Carlos Jr., some of our students, and I represented Rio in some of the Brazilian national wrestling tournaments, and there was always some crooked shit going on. I went to weigh in for the Brazilian championships that were held at the police gymnasium in Rio. A European-looking guy from Minas Gerais they called Salty was in charge, and I was two ounces over weight. When Rolls asked for fifteen minutes for me to cut the weight, Salty slammed his notebook shut and said, "No! He's disqualified."

The referee during the championship match was from Minas Gerais, and he was clearly throwing the match in favor of his fighter. After one especially bad call, my cousin Robson ran onto the mat and slapped the referee in the face. This started a big brawl between our team and the Minas Gerais team. Salty was in the center of the chaos, and I was still pissed off that he had disqualified me, so I punched him in the face. Down he went, just like that. Very quickly, the Minas Gerais team was losing the brawl badly. We chased them out of the gym and down the street, all of us still in our wrestling singlets.

Later we were sued by the wrestling commission, but fortunately one of Rolls's friends filmed everything. After he gave the footage to the sports council, they reviewed it, awarded us the judgment, and dismissed all the cases. In addition to the arbitrary rules, there was another reason why I was losing all interest in wrestling and Sambo. Both sports forced me to reinvent myself as a much more physical fighter who relied on strength and speed rather than intelligence or technique. While Rolls continued to wrestle and tried to establish a Brazilian national team, I was moving toward *vale tudo* because there was little left for me to prove in Jiu Jitsu.

I was growing so dominant in Jiu Jitsu competition that when I stepped onto the mat and the referee said, "Go!" the crowd began to count out loud, "Ten, nine, eight, seven, six . . ." If I didn't submit my opponent in ten seconds, they would start counting again. Even as a black belt, my only Jiu Jitsu fight that went more than five minutes came after the judges robbed my brother Royler of a win against one of my cousin Carlson's students. My final match in the open class was against Carlson's 240-pound heavyweight. I was so upset that I decided that I wanted to make him suffer. After I got him down, I mounted and just put unbearable pressure on him. I was not fighting my actual opponent; instead, I was trying to punish Carlson for robbing Royler.

Everything I was doing was fueled by ego and anger, and I was working against myself because my emotions were negating all of my precision and my martial artistry. I was spinning my wheels as if I were on ice and was going nowhere. I was just blindly punishing him until Rolls yelled, "Eight minutes are up!" I was shocked because that was too long. I snapped to my senses, got mad at myself, and easily submitted him. Afterward, I realized that I never wanted to fight like this again because I was putting emotion before reason. Although nobody else realized it at the time, I learned an important lesson that day—that it was a mistake to fight emotionally because emotions blinded me.

For me, Jiu Jitsu needed to be more like chess—staying many moves ahead of my opponents and using my functional intelligence to take advantage of any windows of opportunity. Rarely are both fighters comfortable in a fight. Almost always, one is applying pressure and one is under pressure. If you are uncomfortable, you are losing. If I am uncomfortable, even for a few seconds, I make the necessary adjustments and get comfortable again. Once I'm comfortable, I'm your worst nightmare. I never knew exactly what an opponent was going to do, but I didn't need to. Once the engagement began, my goal was to use pain and discomfort to force an error, and then checkmate my opponent with a clean submission. As a fighter, despite my progress, I still had homework to do. Now I wanted to use all of the tools I had available in a *vale tudo* fight. I would soon learn that the difference between a Jiu Jitsu match and a *vale tudo* fight was like the difference between kart racing and Formula One.

THE UNFETTERED MIND

HAPPENED TO BE STANDING NEXT TO MY DAD WHEN HIS ONE-time nemesis, Waldemar "the Black Panther" Santana, called him on the phone in 1980. By now, almost thirty years after their legendary three-hour fight, they were friends again and could laugh about it. My dad listened to Waldemar for a while, nodding the entire time, and then turned to me and said, "Waldemar says he has a guy in the north no one can beat. He wants to know if I have a fighter who is up for it. He wants to promote a big event." "Dad! Let me do it! Let me do it!" I begged. Impressed by my enthusiasm, Hélio spoke into the receiver. "Waldemar, I have a boy here who

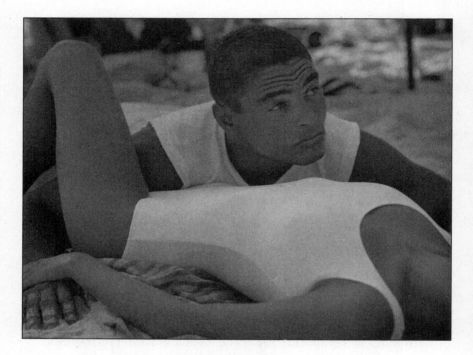

RICKSON AND KIM GRACIE, COPACABANA.
PHOTOGRAPH COURTESY OF BRUCE WEBER.

has never done anything, but I'll take a chance and do the business right. He is my son."

My life at the time was simple. I was nineteen and still living with my parents in the apartment where I grew up. I trained hard every day, made plenty of money teaching, and surfed whenever there were waves. There were big changes on my horizon, though, because in addition to committing to my first professional fight, I had fallen deeply in love.

I had first seen Kim Stavik at the beach and had been struck by her beauty, and besides being a model of physical perfection, she was also an independent woman who was a successful model, a pro surfer, and a pro hang glider. We knew each other by reputation, but the first time we spoke eye to eye and face to face was at a concert at Sugarloaf Mountain. We spent the night together dancing, and there was a strong connection between us. Kim said that she felt as though we had known each other in a past life. Although she was spending more and more nights at my apartment, we also gave each other a great deal of freedom, because she was as active as I was.

Kim would soon see another side of me in my first professional *vale tudo* fight against a massive and terrifying African Brazilian named Casemiro Nascimento Martins, who fought under the stage name King Zulu. He was thirty-three, stood six four, weighed 230 pounds, and supposedly had not lost since 1963. He was not part of a team, an academy, or even an established martial art. He was a dangerous, unorthodox fighter who combined striking with Capoeira footwork and

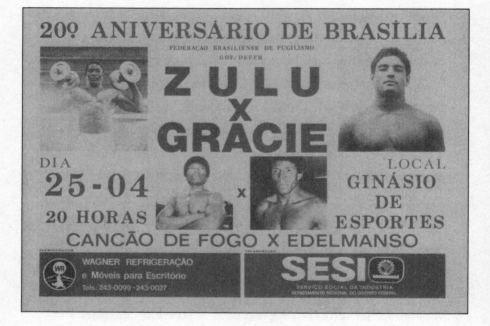

ANNOUNCEMENT FOR RICKSON'S FIRST FIGHT AGAINST KING ZULU.
PHOTOGRAPH COURTESY OF THE RICKSON GRACIE COLLECTION.

grappling. King Zulu also used to like to make faces at his opponents and mock them in the ring.

When my uncle Carlos learned the date of the King Zulu fight, he freaked out and said, "Rickson's emotional, intellectual, and physical biorhythms will be at all-time lows. If I were you, I would postpone the fight." I told my dad that I didn't care about biorhythms or about winning or even losing. I just wanted to test myself. I had been waiting to become a fighter my entire life. No way was I going to back out now.

A month before my fight, my dad and I traveled to Brasília to watch King Zulu fight another giant called Paolo, who made Zulu look small. Because *vale tudo* fighting had been illegal in Rio for many years, I had never been to an actual *vale tudo* fight. The crowd in Brasília was hostile and aggressive, just as I imagine it would have been in the Roman Colosseum. On the sidelines, bookies were giving odds, and spectators were screaming praise and insults at the fighters. There was no pretense of sportsmanship; it was pure madness.

When the fight began, Zulu lifted Paolo all the way over his head and threw him onto the canvas—his trademark move, more reliant on brute strength than technique. The fight ended after King Zulu poked Paolo so hard in the eye that he couldn't continue. Between the raucous crowd and the brutality of the fight, the experience intimidated me. I hoped that Zulu wouldn't throw me on my head, but I figured I was smart enough to avoid it. When I got back to

Rio, I trained with the strongest guys I could find and always started in bad positions like chokes, armlocks, or while mounted. The more uncomfortable, the better.

One month later, my father, Rolls, and I returned to Brasília for the fight. They would be my cornermen. On the day of my fight, Kim, my friends, and other family members arrived. My friend João also came from Rio with a sack full of cash. He went to the stadium with an assistant, who had a notebook, and announced loudly, "I've got money to put on the kid from Rio! I want to bet on the little one! Any takers?" He got a lot of action because King Zulu was undefeated and so much bigger than me. People were practically lining up to place their bets with João.

On the night of the fight, I was stretching in my dressing room with my back to the door when, suddenly, everyone looked toward the door as if a ghost were standing behind me. I felt King Zulu's presence—his looming shadow—but knew that he was trying to rattle me, so I paid no attention to him. Instead, I noticed that the air in Brasília seemed drier than the air in Rio. I remained focused and waited for him to leave. I knew I was ready.

When I finally made my way to the ring, I was struck by the noise. Brazilian sports fans are emotional. I remember someone shouting, "Kill the kid!" I entered the old canvas boxing ring first because King Zulu was already famous and I was just an unknown challenger from Rio. When my opponent got into the ring, he made strange, ugly faces at me and jumped around like a lunatic. This really revved up the crowd. They thought they were about to watch a lamb get fed to a lion.

The bell rang and King Zulu charged across the canvas ring. I held my ground until the last second and threw a brutal knee to his face as he tackled me. Although he took me down, I was sure that I had knocked him out and was thinking about how I would celebrate my first professional victory. Imagine my surprise when King Zulu stood up, shook his head, spat out teeth and blood, and charged again.

When we clinched and started to grapple in the middle of the ring, he put his hand between my legs. I knew that he was trying to set up his trademark throw so I wrapped my leg around one of his so that he couldn't get me off the ground. Then he put his back to the ropes, disentangled my leg—the only thing preventing him from throwing me—and lifted me so high over his head that the bottoms of my feet faced the ceiling. I was now going headfirst toward the concrete ring apron, and the drop was at least eight feet. At the last instant, I was able to grab the top rope, swing my legs underneath me, and land on my feet. I climbed back into the ring, resumed fighting, and finally took him down. When I took his back, I held one of his wrists and elbowed him in the neck. King Zulu was so strong that he crawled out of the ring with me on his back.

I was in shock when the first round ended. I had thrown everything I had at King Zulu, and he was still charging me like an angry bull. I felt I was running out of both gas and options. I got scared. It was like I was looking at a big river that

I needed to cross. Instead of carefully wading in and testing the depth and strength of the current, my mind started telling me, "The other side is too far! The water is too deep! The current is too strong! You can't make it!" I was trying to quit before I had even tried to cross the river. It wasn't until after the fight that I realized how my negative mind-set had intoxicated and filled me with fear and doubt.

When I returned to my corner covered in Zulu's blood, I wondered if it was even possible to hurt this monster. "Throw in the towel! I'm dead," I said to my dad. At first, Hélio just ignored me, then said, "You're doing great! He's more tired than you are." When I said, "No, Dad! I'm serious!" he cut me off and said, "No! He's in much worse shape than you, you're going to kick his ass!" We started arguing and then Rolls dumped a bucket full of ice and water on my head. That shocked me back to my senses, and as I was gasping for breath, the bell rang.

The thought of quitting vanished from my mind as I stepped toward King Zulu. I realized that I had only two options: Kill or die—there was no other way. We were both tired, so the pace of the second round was much slower and less intense. King Zulu threw a big punch that I ducked; then I got him in a clinch. I tried to throw him, and even though I couldn't, it began to dawn on me that my dad was right: King Zulu was more tired than I was. When the crowd saw that the kid from Rio was still standing toe to toe with this killer, the momentum shifted in my direction. Everyone loves an underdog, and now people were yelling, "C'mon kid! You can do it!"

After struggling for a bit on our feet, I eventually wrestled King Zulu to the ground, immediately took his back, and began to elbow him in the head and back of the neck. Then I sunk a choke, and what had been hell just three minutes before turned to pure bliss. When I won, the crowd was stunned.

Moments after my win, Zulu hugged me and said, "Kid, congratulations, but you've got all that help, and I'm a self-made fighter." I hugged him back and thanked him for the opportunity to fight.

My friend and adviser Sergio Zveiter had also come to Brasília to support me. Prior to the fight, he'd had some doubts that he did not express until later. After I won, Sergio was overjoyed, not because I won but because I had showed him the power and possibilities that Jiu Jitsu gave you. This reinforced his belief that if I could beat King Zulu, he too was capable of anything. Later Uncle Carlos said to me, "If you were able to do that at the worst possible biorhythmic time, imagine what you can do at your best!" Kim was also impressed because I think it was the first time she realized what it meant to be a Gracie.

Once the celebrations were over, I had to face the fact that this was the toughest experience of my life and that my father and brother were the keys to my victory. They had brought me back from a full panic attack. This also had made me realize how much I had to thank my family for. My measure of a brave man, a true fighter, is not how many times he gets knocked down, but how many times he gets back up.

Even today, I am grateful to King Zulu for making me into a much better fighter.

This fight exposed me to the most primal kind of fear that comes from within. My insecure state of mind came from the fear of losing. If you fear something that has not even happened, then quitting becomes a form of self-protection. Fear is not the enemy; it's simply a self-protection mechanism that must be managed.

At the time, I was not confident enough to believe in myself unconditionally and was afraid of the unknown. It was a terrible feeling. Although my dad and brother pushed me through it, I reminded myself that doubts and an insecure state of mind would cripple me as a fighter. I realized that if I could control my mind, I could improve every aspect of my performance. If you have this kind of spiritual security, you realize that physicality is only one part of the puzzle.

Everything had been theoretical up to now, but now I was faced with new realities. My first *vale tudo* fight taught me that sometimes you don't break physically but emotionally. Although I was already physically and mentally confident, I wasn't spiritually and emotionally confident. If you don't have the spiritual connection, you can't dance on the razor's edge. I made a vow to myself that from that day forward I would always try to cross the river no matter the consequences. This made a huge difference, not just in my fighting career, but in the way I looked at life. Moving forward, if I committed to something, I was resigned to the outcome no matter what it might be.

I had always been looking for things that could help me grow as an athlete, but now I was truly hungry for this knowledge. I knew that if my dad and Rolls hadn't been in my corner, I would've quit. If I was to become the greatest Gracie, I couldn't rely on others. I was the only one who would step into that ring, take on that responsibility, and uphold that honor.

My mother, ever so patient, was always trying to find ways to give me peace of mind. First she tried to get me into yoga, but I found the positions and postures painful and unnatural. Next she took me to Transcendental Meditation, but when I chanted my mantra, I either fell asleep or couldn't concentrate well enough to do it. A gymnast friend, who knew a great deal about yoga, told me about a guy named Orlando Cani, who was developing a system of movement that one day would be called Bioginástica. Cani's goal was to get people to move and breathe like animals in order to rediscover their natural instincts. Instead of being intelligent and rational, he wanted his students to become sensitive and intuitive.

Orlando Cani believed that modern man had become disconnected from his body because he had been taught to think instead of feel. Most people assume that there is a clear dividing line between the mind and body, but there isn't. Their relationship is much more symbiotic and complex. He tried to reestablish the mind-body connection by making his students conscious of their everyday movements, things like getting out of bed, walking, and climbing ladders. This complex simplicity spoke to me because it was so much like Jiu Jitsu.

My first class was a basic group class that Orlando asked me to take so he could evaluate me. When I walked into his studio, I saw an altar with a Buddha on it surrounded by some offerings. The floors were hardwood; there were mirrors on one side and floor-to-ceiling ladders on the other. My classmates were about a dozen men and women aged twenty-five to fifty, regular people of all levels of fitness and coordination.

Although Orlando Cani looked like a 1970s hippie yoga teacher, nothing could have been further from the truth. Two decades my senior, he was a former paratrooper and one of the greatest athletes in Brazilian history. A champion swimmer, gymnast, runner, and marksman, Cani was also proficient in a number of martial arts. After he won his second world military pentathlon, the president of Brazil, Humberto Castelo Branco, awarded him the nation's highest athletic honor, the Sport Cross of Merit. After retiring from competition, he turned his full attention to Hatha-yoga and Pranayama breathing, and he traveled to India to study with Shri Yogendra, the father of modern yoga.

When the class began, I was immediately impressed by Orlando Cani's agility and how well he moved for his age. We followed and tried to copy his movements as he talked to us and encouraged the class to relax, breathe, and empty our minds. He would say, "Imagine you are a bird, move your arms." This was rhythmic and flowing, like dance and unlike yoga; I found it easy to slip into a more meditative state of mind. I wasn't thinking, I was just following Orlando and copying his movements. Toward the end of the class, he took me aside and said, "Rickson, you're special. I want to teach you privately because your ability level is so high."

Cani's classes were not for everyone. You did not go to his studio to lose weight or to build muscles. Many students were confused by his commands because he would never say, "Do ten more reps." Instead he would say, "Extend your body's trunk, maintain neck posture, exhale, and let your internal energy flow." If you are moving and breathing, you can't have other thoughts in your head. You can't think, then move and breathe; it's not the same. He wanted to focus on the body's "psychomotor system" in order to develop fast, smooth, and explosive extension and flexibility.

First I learned the basic postures and the type of breathing that went with each one. Once I could do these correctly, he incorporated movement and martial arts animal forms. Ancient Kung Fu masters choreographed postures and movements based on the ways different animals move and fight. The tiger combines strength with mobility and attacks forcefully and directly. The crane is evasive, graceful, and relies on its long neck and sharp beak for both offense and defense. The snake is fast, agile, and deceptive and can both strike and strangle. Orlando liked us to try to emulate different animals because they use their strength and flexibility naturally.

In a relatively short time, I was able to combine breathing with fast movement and enter into a meditative state.

One day, Orlando Cani started class and the phone rang. He had to take the call and told me to continue without him. For the first time, I was not playing follow the leader. I started to breathe and move and breathe and move and quickly got lost in the motion. I was jumping from ladder to ladder like a monkey. At one point, I almost felt that I could fly. All of my movements, whether standing, climbing, or on the ground, were flowing, and my transitions were seamless. I was completely unconscious.

When I came back to my senses, I was on the highest rung on the ladder, dripping with sweat. I looked around and saw Orlando Cani in the corner crying. I asked my teacher what was going on. He said, "I have nothing left to teach you."

I asked him how he could say that, and he said, "I've been watching you for the last hour and ten minutes. I called to you a few times, and you didn't hear me; you kept moving. You were in a total meditative state; your brain and consciousness were completely turned off." It was an emotional moment for both of us.

Whenever I entered this empty-mind state, I could neither hear nor talk and was not conscious of my movements. Not only did my mind go blank, but afterward I felt as if my brain had been cleaned and reset. This gave me the ability to retreat from my own consciousness and come back stronger. I noticed the effects immediately. I was able to focus with absolute clarity and my senses grew sharper, as did my awareness of my body and surroundings.

By far the most important thing that Orlando Cani taught

me was how to control my breathing. You can go weeks without food and days without water, but five minutes without air and you're dead. Think about that for a minute. These breathing techniques would become especially important in the coming years, because they made it much easier for me to gauge and control fear, adrenaline, panic, and claustrophobia. For example, if I want to control my adrenaline when I'm nervous, I breathe at a slower pace until I get my emotions under control. If I want to increase my pace, I don't use my mind to tell my body to speed up; I just breathe deeper and faster. During high exertion, exhaling becomes more important than inhaling. To enjoy a good deep breath, you must consciously empty your lungs.

When I breathe with my belly, I get more oxygen and expel more carbon dioxide. Not knowing how to breathe is like having a hand and not knowing how to use your fingers! Most people are chest breathers, meaning that their stomach does not move when they breathe because they don't use their diaphragm, only the upper part of their lungs. If you breathe from your chest, the breaths are short and panicky.

One of the most important muscles for high-performance athletes to develop in order to breathe more efficiently is the diaphragm. Cani realized that a person breathing normally uses less than 50 percent of the lungs' capacity, so he applied Pranayama techniques to athletics and was able to utilize 80 percent of the lungs' capacity. This conscious approach to breathing is just like using the different gears of a car's transmission. Flutists, opera singers, snipers, divers, and big-wave surfers all understand the importance of breathing. To-day, you hear the top tennis pros screaming "Ahh" when they hit the ball, because they know that the forceful exhalation gives them speed and more explosive power.

Everything I have earned today was at least partially a result of breathing—my best performance, my emotional control, my ability to endure. Breathing gave me all of this.

Once I started to learn the mechanics of breathing and how to apply them, my sprint became twice as long as my opponent's sprint, yet my recovery time was three to four times faster. I learned that if my opponent's heart rate was at 80 to 90 beats per minute (bpm) and mine was 60, in no time he would be at 120 bpm while I'd be only at 90. Soon he'd be at 150 and I'd still only be at 100 bpm. That was when his panic would set in—when he realized that he needed a break and I didn't.

Orlando Cani taught me how to empty my mind and use intuition instead of my brain. After training with him, my perception improved to the point where I could shake some-one's hand and instantly determine if he was friend or foe, re-laxed or tense, happy or sad, confident or insecure. This gave me a huge advantage in the ring. When I fought, I was neither emotional nor intellectual. I never thought about strategy; I just allowed myself to connect with my opponent on a pro-found level. The moment the bell rang, I didn't expect any-thing or plan anything. In order to do this, I had to rid myself of all thoughts about victory or defeat. Anything I didn't need

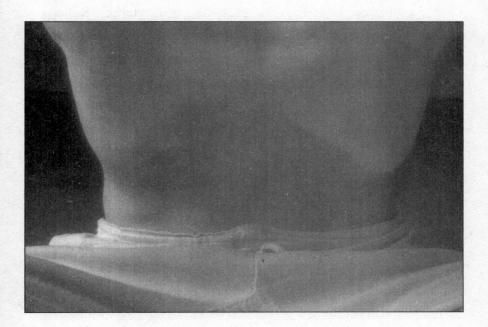

RICKSON GRACIE, RIO DE JANEIRO, 1988.
PHOTOGRAPH COURTESY OF MARCOS PRADO / @REVISTATRIP, 1988.

for that specific fight against that specific opponent went on the shelf.

I soon field-tested these principles on the mat and in the ring. I would learn to bring my fights to a boiling point, and when my opponent needed to rest, I would turn up the heat and go for the kill. With the exception of my father, Hélio, and my brother Rolls, Orlando Cani was the most important teacher of my life. He helped me to see fighting through a more spiritual and emotional lens. Once I could accept death and walk comfortably toward it, what was there to be afraid of? My biggest personal breakthrough came after realizing that my life was less important than my mission. I was always courageous but would often waste my courage on stupid things that put me at unnecessary risk. For example, I was fine with risking my life in big surf because I felt that it helped me grow, but going to a party and getting into a fight now seemed stupid and even reckless. I wanted to calculate my risks and save them for things that would advance my mission to become the greatest Gracie.

While I admired the soccer player Pelé, the swimmer Mark Spitz, and a handful of other great athletes, I was inspired most by the greatest Brazilian race car driver of all time, Ayrton Senna. We were roughly the same age, and there were many similarities in our training methodology and outlook on competition. We both believed that the harder you trained, the easier you raced or fought. When Senna's races were canceled due to rain, he would take his car out and practice in the worst possible conditions. In 1984, during his rookie season, the Monaco Grand Prix was held in a massive rainstorm. World champions were spinning out and crashing, but Senna, an unknown rookie in a shitty car, drove better and faster than all of them. He once said that when he was driving a car at the limit of its performance envelope, he was not conscious of driving. That was exactly how I felt when I was fighting.

I don't think it's a coincidence that Ayrton Senna was also a selfless and deeply spiritual man. Even though he was notoriously competitive, he also had great compassion. During a practice session for the 1992 Belgian Grand Prix, French driver Érik Comas crashed into a barrier at two hundred miles per hour and was knocked unconscious. When Senna drove up to the crash, he could hear the Frenchman's engine revving at redline and realized that Comas's foot was still on the accelerator of the crashed car and that it could burst into flames at any moment. Without a second's hesitation, Senna stopped in the middle of the track, jumped out of his car, sprinted over to Comas, shut down the motor, and stabilized the driver's neck until the ambulance arrived. I was sad, but not surprised, when Senna died on the racetrack in 1994. He had been operating on the razor's edge for quite some time by then.

After training with Orlando, I was willing to fight anyone under any rules. I didn't care if he was two hundred pounds heavier than me. It was a particular kind of suicide, but I was willing to sacrifice my body to achieve my larger mission. Now I visualized my worst nightmares with spiritual comfort, not fear. If I had to die in the process, well fuck, then die I had to.

In addition to the mental advances that I was making, my relationship with Kim had gotten serious, and this marked a big step forward for me in my relationships with women. I didn't see Kim as just another girl; I wanted to have a relationship with her because I felt like I had met my mate. She was independent, strong, beautiful, and had a good sense of humor. And Kim was not a party girl who had to have perfect clothes and makeup all of the time. She could surf and spend the day at the beach. Kim liked great restaurants, but she was also content with simple things like eating a good meal at home. For a time, we really complemented each other and were living the dream. I gave her a sense of security that she had never had, and she encouraged me to think big. She was everything I wanted in a woman, and I felt that I had met my perfect match.

I was ecstatic when Kim got pregnant with our first son, Rockson. Though we weren't planning on having kids so soon, I knew that she loved me and that she knew how important family was to me. I had no conception of life without one. For her it was more difficult, because she was a model and a pro surfer; a child would have a big impact on her career aspirations. Nonetheless, Kim's pregnancy was a beautiful time in our lives.

When Kim went into labor, we went to a small clinic in Rio for her to give birth. Her labor was long, and I was standing behind her when Rockson squirmed into the doctor's hands. When I saw his dick, it was the happiest day of my life. I loved that baby more than I loved myself. Fourteen hours later the three of us were home at our apartment, and I was starting a new chapter in my life.

Rockson was not an easy baby. He didn't sleep much and he cried all the time. When we got home from the hospital, I was up all night with him so Kim could recover. My son was born on Tuesday, and I went Wednesday, Thursday, and Friday without sleeping much, or training. That Sunday, however, I was in the finals of a Jiu Jitsu competition against Sérgio Penha. At that time, Penha was the latest Jiu Jitsu phenom who had won everything and skyrocketed to the top of the food chain.

This tournament took place on two consecutive weekends, and I had already defeated him the previous weekend. Initially, I was going to fight in the middleweight division, but when I saw that Penha was a heavyweight, I told the tournament organizer, "Let's make this a real party. Put me in the heavyweight division." On the first Sunday, we faced off in the heavyweight division, and I made him tap after catching him in an armlock. He had not been finished that quickly in many years and was out for revenge when we met in the open division finals the next Sunday.

When our fight started and we engaged, I felt weak and my recovery was off. I pretended to fight but was really just conserving my energy for one opportunity. When we went to the ground, Sérgio passed my guard, which made the crowd go crazy. I was down by 7 or 8 points in a matter of seconds.

I pretended to be dead and let my opponent gain confidence. The crowd thought that they were about to witness the greatest upset in Jiu Jitsu history! People wanted to see the underdog win and were screaming, "Believe, Sérgio! Courage, Sérgio!" Toward the end of the fight, Sergio was ahead on points 15–0. I turned to Rolls and asked, "How much time?" When he said two minutes, I knew that it was now or never. I pulled guard and when he tried to pass, I reversed him, took the side, mounted, and put him in a collar choke. Sérgio was a valiant guy; he didn't tap, and I put him to sleep with forty-five seconds remaining.

Jiu Jitsu tournaments were getting less and less interesting to me. Rockson's birth forced me to look beyond Jiu Jitsu and think about what kind of family I wanted, as well as to take a harder look at the one I was born into. Hélio was almost seventy when Rockson was born, and his mind-set was still straight out of the 1950s. He didn't care if his grandsons were educated or polite, so long as they were good soldiers for his army. Hélio would always acknowledge Carlos Gracie, the clan, and the universe, but he could never recognize my mother for the support that she gave him. Growing up, I felt that my mother was always sad. Sometimes I would find her crying and ask, "Mother, what's wrong?" Even though she would always say that nothing was, I realized that she was quietly suffering. I saw how much she sacrificed for my father and her kids—and how little my dad reciprocated or even acknowledged it. Can you imagine being married to Hélio Gracie?

While there were many things I liked about the Gracie traditions, polygamy was not one of them. Uncle Carlos and Hélio were not the first polygamous Gracies. Their father, Gastão, had five children with another woman while he was married to my grandmother. I was about thirteen when my father asked me, "Would you like to have more brothers?" I said yes and he told me to get in the car. We drove to an apartment building in Botafogo, about ten minutes away, and took the elevator to the sixth floor. Hélio knocked on one of the doors. It was cracked open, and Vera, a woman who worked at the academy, stuck her head out the top. Then one little head popped out the bottom of the crack and smiled at me, then another, and then another. "They're all your brothers," my dad said. That was the first time I met my brothers Rolker, Royler, and Royce. The kids were cute and friendly, but as much as I liked them, I couldn't help but feel sorry for my mom. My father never told her that he wanted more children. He just showed up one day with four more! At first mom was depressed, but eventually Hélio convinced her to become friends with Vera. Although my mother pretended to move on, I could see how much this hurt her.

Once I became a parent, I saw that my dad and Uncle Carlos were dinosaurs, that their outlook and their relationships were all static and frozen in time. This tempered my admiration for them, and I didn't want to be that way. My wife, Kim, supported me wholeheartedly, and I recognized that without her help, I would not have made it as far as I did. I saw the sacrifices she made for me, how she was always willing to put me first and herself second. My dad would never have appreciated his wife like that; he didn't give a fuck about how my mother felt. In Hélio Gracie's mind, his mission was bigger than these kinds of sensitivities.

The year 1982 was a bittersweet one. I was now the father of the son I had always dreamed of, but I also suffered a devastating loss. In June, Rolls and his family went to Maua for a family weekend in the mountains. Rolls noticed that his old hang glider was strapped to the roof of a car in front of his hotel. It turned out that the owner was a friend of a friend. Even though my brother had promised his wife, Angela, that he would quit hang gliding after he'd had several close calls and friends had died in accidents, he made arrangements to go the next day.

The following day, the conditions were very bad because there was no wind. If Rolls got his mind set on something, however, there was no saying no to him. Although the owner of his old hang glider did not want to go because he thought it was too dangerous, Rolls talked him into letting him use it for just one flight.

My brother ran down the ramp, launched, initially got some lift but then began to spiral, and he hit the ground ninety yards from the ramp. His friend ran into the overgrown forest and found my brother hanging upside down with his eyes wide open. Although he looked perfectly fine, his neck was broken, and Rolls was dead.

I received the news over the phone, and it took only seconds to know that my life would never be the same. Not only had I lost an idol, a teacher, and my favorite brother, but I was now the official family champion. Now I would have to answer all the challenges and lead the next generation of Gracie fighters. I was now my family's last line of defense.

Rolls's funeral was held in a cemetery near downtown. All of our family was there except for Uncle Carlos, who was too devastated to attend. Inside the casket, Rolls was dressed in a T-shirt and looked normal except for his neck, which was very swollen. Sadly, this was my very last image of him. I missed him then, and I still miss him today. His death affected our family dynamics dramatically. Rolls had brought the two sides together because he was Carlos's son, but was raised by Hélio. He had acted as a bridge between the two sides of the family, but now that bridge was gone forever.

STEEL SHARPENS STEEL

THE FIRST SIGNIFICANT SPLIT IN THE FAMILY CAME WHEN IT WAS time for Rolls's widow, Angela, to decide who would take over his academy. Although my father wanted it, she gave it to Rolls's brother Carlos Jr. instead, and he would soon emerge as my father's biggest Jiu Jitsu rival. While Hélio was content to continue teaching Jiu Jitsu as a self-defense martial art, Carlos Jr. had big ideas about how to transform it into a competitive sport with standardized rules, sponsors, and officially sanctioned tournaments with referees and time limits.

After my fight with King Zulu, I was growing less interested in Jiu Jitsu and more so in *vale tudo*. In 1983, the media conglomerate Grupo Globo was trying to promote the South American boxing championship at the Maracanãzinho Gymnasium in Rio. They included one *vale tudo* fight and announced that King Zulu was coming down from the north and issuing a challenge to Rio's fighters. This was a big deal, because *vale tudo* fights had been banned in Rio for decades.

At first I wasn't that interested in fighting King Zulu because I had already beaten him. Above all, I was curious to see who would step up and accept the challenge. I was hoping that a tough Luta Livre fighter like Denilson Maia or a kickboxer like Flávio Molina might answer the call. Someone had to defend Rio's honor, and there were plenty of fighters who could. I figured that it was just a matter of time before one of them announced that he was fighting Zulu.

Three weeks later . . . silence. Not one fighter from Rio stepped forward! It was like a giant swell had hit the coast and everyone was pretending that there were no waves because they were afraid to paddle out. I understand why most fighters at the time were scared—*vale tudo* was unknown territory. A *vale tudo* match is not a Jiu Jitsu tournament or a kickboxing bout. Those who fight ten-minute rounds without gloves, mouthpiece, or cup—win or lose—will leave their comfort zone.

Finally, the promoters came directly to me and asked me to fight King Zulu again for the princely sum of maybe $5,000. After I accepted the challenge, the event sold out the seventeen-thousand-seat stadium. This time I had a home-court advantage because the fight would be at Maracanãzinho

Gymnasium, where my father had fought Kimura, and all of my friends, family, and students would be there.

The night of the fight, the stadium was packed with a very loud and rowdy crowd. In our first fight, King Zulu was reckless because he didn't fear or respect me. In our second fight, he was much more careful and did not charge me when the bell rang. When we finally connected in a clinch, he picked me up and slammed me but wound up in my guard. Thanks to Orlando Cani, mentally I was a different fighter now. In this fight, I was confident and prepared, and my body was on autopilot. At a certain point, a fight becomes a transcendental experience. It was as if I was in the wheelhouse of a ship at sea looking out of a porthole at the chaos of a stormy sea all around me. I had been here before and my body needed no instructions.

Even with King Zulu inside my guard trying to head-butt me and gouge my eyes, I was totally calm. This time I felt that my opponent was fighting much more cautiously and it would take me time to cook him down. I stayed on my back, made sure to control his head, and heel-kicked him over and over in the kidneys and floating ribs. He survived the first round by staying calm inside my guard and didn't make a mistake. I was in no hurry. I knew that King Zulu was burning far more energy than I was.

It was so loud when the second round began that I could not hear the bell. Meanwhile, King Zulu was trying to get inside of my head by filling his cheeks with air, making faces at me, and jumping around the ring. I still was not sure if the

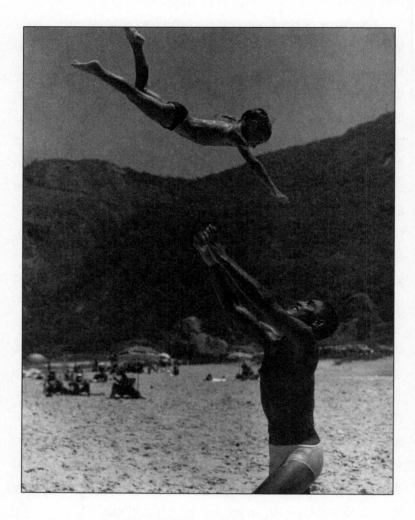

RICKSON AND ROCKSON GRACIE, COPACABANA.
PHOTOGRAPH COURTESY OF BRUCE WEBER.

round had started so I turned to the referee and held both of my thumbs up. When he nodded yes, I attacked; we clinched and went to the ground. He tried to grab my neck, but I was able to slip out of his hold and take his back. As I began to sink my choke, I felt my opponent's gigantic fingers crawling around on my face, trying to find an eye to gouge, but it was too late and I submitted him with a choke. King Zulu never got exhausted as he did in our first fight. He just made that one mistake.

What would have stressed me before I trained with Orlando Cani was now child's play. My potential was not growing a little bit; it was growing by leaps and bounds. I now felt as though I had a reserve parachute that nobody else had, and I was ready for anything. Winning the rematch with Zulu in Rio established me as the *vale tudo* champion to beat.

Not much changed in my day-to-day life. I kept teaching, training, competing in Jiu Jitsu, and raising my son. I was convinced that he was going to be just like me. Even as a tiny child, Rockson was intense, incredibly coordinated, focused, and nimble. As he grew, I tried to make him as athletic and fearless as possible. I threw him into the air as my father had done with me, and then bought him a trampoline that he would bounce on for hours. I also encouraged him to hang on ropes for as long as possible.

At twenty-one, I was a young father, and I gave Rockson everything a boy could ever want. For example, when he was just a small child, I bought him a brand-new surfboard. Today, I would say, "If you want that surfboard, you have to be nicer to your mother. You have to put your clothes in the drawer and peel all the apples for a week, and then I will get you one." Many years later, I realized that things mean more if you earn them, but when I was young and wanted to give him a present, I didn't think twice.

Rockson's birth did not change the way I led my day-to-day life. I left our apartment at seven in the morning and taught and trained until ten at night. I could still go to the beach in the middle of the day and surf with my friends and do many other things that my wife could no longer do. Kim began to get frustrated, and for the first time, some friction began to enter our relationship. Children alter the course of a relationship because the focus is no longer on the two partners. I was young and craved the passion with Kim that we once had. I started to drift away and have casual affairs with other women. I never disrespected Kim by rubbing her face in it, but she had a sixth sense and knew something was up. She began to grow colder toward me, and I grew more distant as a result. Still, we both loved Rockson and remained united in our mission to raise him.

I had another distraction when the Luta Livre challenges began. Luta Livre is a no-gi style of grappling and *vale tudo* fighting that had been around for many years. A wrestler named Euclydes "Tatu" Hatem created the style in the 1920s and fought my uncle George in the 1940s. By the 1980s, Tatu's student Fausto Brunocilla and his son Carlos had taken over and had a number of tough students, like Marco Ruas,

Hugo Duarte, and Eugenio Tadeu, who would go on to make names for themselves in the early years of MMA.

Although the Luta Livre fighters had been our rivals for decades, things between us had escalated before Rolls died, when a karate fighter sucker-punched one of my younger cousins on the street. My cousin was just a kid, and the other guy was an adult. When Rolls heard about this, he went straight down to his teacher Flávio Molina's Naja Academy, and a huge brawl broke out.

After that, Molina, who was one of Brazil's first Thai boxers, started to practice grappling with the Luta Livre fighters to be better prepared against Jiu Jitsu fighters. Rather than brawl in the street, we decided to settle the score in the ring with a *vale tudo* tournament between Jiu Jitsu and Luta Livre. Jiu Jitsu was represented by my student Marcelo Behring, Fernando Pinduka, and Renan Pitanguy; representing Luta Livre were Marco Ruas, Eugênio Tadeu, and Flávio Molina. The fights were very tough, and in the end, Jiu Jitsu won one, lost one, and tied one. The Luta Livre guys were happy with their performance. By cross-training with kickboxers like Molina, some of the Luta Livre fighters were beginning to feel and act as if they had figured out a formula to beat Jiu Jitsu.

Although my and Kim's relationship remained tense, she got pregnant again and had our second child in 1984, a beautiful baby girl we named Kauan. Unlike Rockson, who was intense, Kauan was peaceful and happy. She smiled constantly and was strong, steady, and calm like a little Buddha. Everybody wanted to hold her and hug her. She loved Rockson and looked up to him, but was not as coordinated as he. Kauan would try to emulate him—her spirit was willing—but we had to watch out for her because she would sometimes hurt herself trying to keep up with him. Kauan's real gifts were artistic; she loved music, singing, and dancing. Anytime we put music on, she would start to dance.

Though Kauan was a very positive addition to our family, Kim's resentment of me continued to grow. Now she had two small children to take care of, and I still had not changed my ways. I was gone training and teaching most of the time. As much as she loved our children, motherhood was a hard transition for her. In the blink of an eye, she had gone from a model with the world at her feet to a mother at home with two babies. While I am not proud of it today, truth be told, I was young, famous, and selfish. The most beautiful women in Rio were throwing themselves at me, and the fact that I did not always resist the temptations did not help matters.

Whatever happened between Kim and me, I was never going to leave my children in the wind. They were too important. In order for me to be happy, I had to be with my kids. I wanted to teach them about respect and honesty. What if Kim remarried a guy who drank, smoked, and was a bad influence on them? Despite my failings as a husband and our fighting, I knew that Kim loved our kids more than anything and took very good care of them. We still loved each other and tried to make our marriage work, but I had a limited and unusual frame of reference when it came to women and relationships. Carlos and Hélio Gracie were not exactly sensitive New Age guys, and some of their attitude had obviously rubbed off on me.

In 1986, Kim gave birth to our third child, a second daughter we named Kaulin, who was more like Rockson than her older sister. Even though she was shy, Kaulin was curious and not afraid of anything. She was a warrior who imposed her will and did things her way.

Despite the strains in our marriage, my children brought me great joy. When American fashion photographer Bruce Weber came to Rio to take pictures of Brazilian athletes in 1986, he heard about me. After we met at his hotel and talked for a while, he became fascinated by my family and interested in our history and traditions. The way that Bruce works is informal and very intimate. Because he wanted to understand me, he went to the beach with us, ate meals with us, and closely observed how we lived and raised our kids. His photographs brought us to life because they showed that although I was one of the toughest people on earth, I was still a human—playful, gentle, and caring with my children. Bruce intuitively understood the complexity of my life and personality. We became friends and still are to this day. Not only did Bruce Weber take some beautiful pictures, but he was really the first person to introduce me to an international audience. It was not hard for us to pretend to be the perfect family: Kim and our children were beautiful, I was a successful athlete, and from the outside our family looked ideal. The truth was less kind.

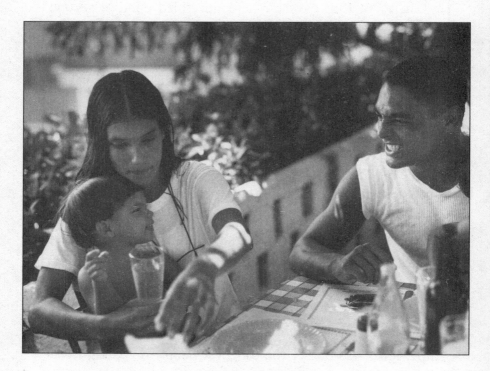

KAUAN, KIM, AND RICKSON GRACIE, RIO.
PHOTOGRAPH COURTESY OF BRUCE WEBER.

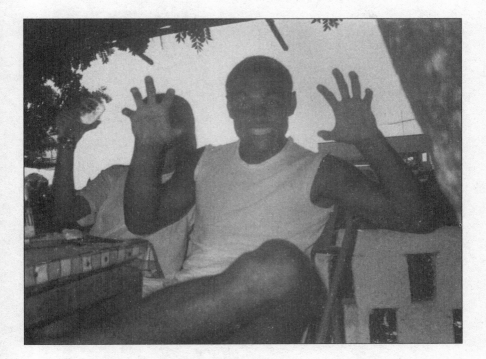

RICKSON GRACIE.
PHOTOGRAPH COURTESY OF BRUCE WEBER.

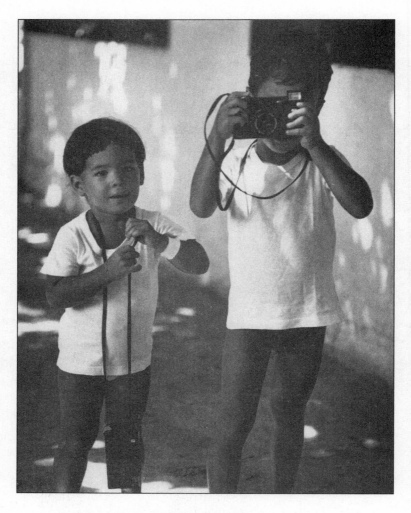

KAUAN AND ROCKSON GRACIE, RIO DE JANEIRO, 1988.
PHOTOGRAPH COURTESY OF BRUCE WEBER.

The Gracie clan continued to divide along bloodlines. While Rorion was trying to establish our martial art in the United States, Carlos Gracie Jr. was going in a different direction in Brazil and primarily focusing on a competitive form of Jiu Jitsu that would come to be known as sport Jiu Jitsu. Carlos was a smart and creative guy, but behind closed doors, he and I always argued. He thought that because the Gracie family was already famous, all we needed to do was maintain our reputation. Carlos always wanted to lead, but never did the kind of heavy lifting that I did. I didn't inherit the title of family champion. I earned it with blood, sweat, and tears.

Carlos deserves much of the credit for creating sport Jiu Jitsu, but with it came a problem. It transformed our martial art and created a lot of paper tigers who would never step into the ring to carry the flag of Gracie Jiu Jitsu. My father didn't like the sport version because he thought that it was watering down our martial art. Hélio used to say, "This is not my Jiu Jitsu, because competitive Jiu Jitsu is not a martial art. The Jiu Jitsu I created is a martial art so a person can defend themselves on the street without getting beaten up."

Just how much things were changing became clear to me during one of my last big tournaments, in Rio in 1986. I was surprised to see that Carlos Gracie Jr. had my cousins Rigan Machado and Jean Jacques Machado listed as his students. I had not trained with the Machado brothers in a while, but they were also my students. Rigan was a big, skilled black belt who had won the Brazilian national championship every year at every belt. Like me, Rigan had not lost a tournament match since he was fourteen.

I was even more surprised when Carlos claimed that the sponsor demanded a match between me and my cousin. I didn't believe him. Rigan was Carlos's first black belt and one of the family's rising stars. If he beat me, he would be the new king of Gracie Jiu Jitsu. The sponsorship thing was bullshit. Carlos had been whispering in Rigan's ear: "Imagine if you win. You'll be the new family champion."

When Carlos told me about the match, I told him, "Carlos, you're making a mistake by having me fight Rigan and breaking our family alliance over a fucking sponsor." I hadn't trained with the Machado brothers in a while; maybe Rigan thought that he could beat me now, so I warned both of them that if we fought, I would not hold back.

When we faced off in the open-class final, we engaged, and Rigan threw me hard onto the mat. I recovered, swept him, and we went back and forth at full speed. Both of us had our gas pedals floored, and although my cousin was bigger, I knew that he could not keep pace with me. With three minutes left, he was exhausted by the pace and intensity, and I caught him in a choke. After the fight, Rigan came to me and said, "Fighting you was the worst mistake I've ever made in my life. I never want to fight you again. I did this because Carlos asked me to."

"No problem. Let's forget about it."

I had little interest in the politics of Jiu Jitsu, and I had three children to support. I wanted to fight *vale tudo* professionally, and the only place to do it outside of Brazil was Japan. Fighting in Japan was not that simple, because the yakuza, the powerful Japanese organized crime syndicates, were heavily involved in almost all of the fight promotions. Worse, many of the fighters were pro wrestlers, and although they were large, strong, and skilled, many of their fights were "works," or fixed fights. I refused to do fixed fights. I traveled to Japan with my friend and informal adviser Sergio Zveiter for the first time in 1987 with a letter of introduction to Antonio Inoki, a former wrestler who had fought a demonstration bout with Muhammad Ali in 1976. By now, he had retired from the ring and had become one of Japan's most powerful fight promoters.

Even before I went there, Japan had always been a part of my life. Jiu Jitsu is Japanese, and I knew that my uncle had learned it from a Japanese fighter and heard about my dad's fights against Japanese fighters. I don't believe in coincidences and think the connection is much deeper than that. Why was my dad the most prominent Jiu Jitsu fighter and teacher in Brazil? Why did generation after generation of my family learn Jiu Jitsu and fight to prove its efficiency and superiority? When I was a young boy, I even had dreams in which I spoke fluent Japanese. I understood what I was saying and even remember having an argument in one of them. However, when I woke up in Rio, I could no longer understand the language.

Inoki would not see me immediately, so while I was waiting I explored Tokyo. First, I went to the Kōdōkan, the world's most famous Judo school, to pay my respects. This was where Judo's inventor and founder, Jigarō Kanō, taught Hideyo Maeda, who in turn taught my uncles. I felt obliged to go there, given what Maeda had done for my family. Although the Kōdōkan's Judo masters welcomed me with open arms, when I told them that I was in Japan to set up a pro fight, they politely told me that I could not train there. Jigarō Kanō did not allow prize fighting.

After much waiting and even more formalities, Inoki refused to meet with me. In the end, his organization wanted me to be one of their stable fighters, like a pro wrestler. To him I probably looked like just another unknown fighter looking for his big break. Even though the trip seemed like a waste of time, it taught me things about Japan that would help me in the coming years.

First, I learned how structured a society it was and how rules and hierarchies were respected more than anything else. Second, I learned the importance of unquestioning obedience. The number-two man never questions the number-one man, no matter how wrong he is. To me, following someone who you knew was wrong was beyond reason or honor; it was just blind obedience. This also made me reevaluate my view of the samurai. According to the samurai code of Bushido (the code of the warrior), honor and loyalty were more important than wealth, life, and family. On the battlefield, the samurai had absolute loyalty and courage and were great warriors, but they did not fight for themselves. The samurai were servants from their first day to their last, because they were bound by honor to stick with their master. The word *samurai* actually means "one who serves," and his only dreams and ambitions were to be those of his shogun.

After I failed to get a fight in Japan, I returned to Brazil, and my dad began trying to convince me to move to California to help Rorion promote Gracie Jiu Jitsu there. My dad convinced me that Rorion needed the best Gracies in the US to help him spread the martial art. This made sense to me, but I didn't want to leave my family behind. Things at home grew even more strained when Kim got pregnant with our fourth child. It was a very difficult pregnancy; she had to remain in bed for most of it, or she risked losing the baby. One day Kim exploded at me, and all of her resentment for me and her present situation boiled over. After she said some harsh things to me in the heat of the moment, I said, "If you're not happy with me here, I'm going to live at my friend's house. I'll come by to see the kids and will give you all the support you need."

Even though I regained my freedom, now that I had kids, it didn't feel the same. When my second son, Kron, was born, Kim and I were still separated. Kron was a calm baby, completely different from Rockson. He smiled all the time and had a very good sense of humor. We called him *bozinho*, which means "a good one" in Portuguese. The girls smothered him with affection, but Kim was adamant that my relationship with him was not going to be like my relationship with Rockson. Even at seven years old, Rockson was

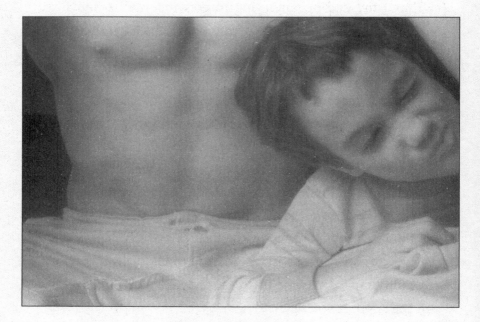

RICKSON AND ROCKSON GRACIE, RIO DE JANEIRO, 1988.
PHOTOGRAPH COURTESY OF MARCOS PRADO / @REVISTATRIP, 1988.

my right-hand man and went everywhere with me. He was already intent on being a Gracie and a fighter.

Once people heard that I was leaving for America, a rumor started to circulate that Marco Ruas, one of Luta Livre's best fighters (who would go on to become a UFC champion), wanted to fight me. I could not officially challenge Ruas, because I was the champion and an established name and Ruas had only fought my student to a draw. While I didn't want to challenge him, I needed to show that I was willing to fight him anytime, anywhere.

One evening my father, Marcelo Behring, Sergio Zveiter, and I drove over to the Luta Livre academy. We walked in and twenty or thirty fighters stopped training and stared at us. Marco Ruas walked over, and greeted us. Everyone was very respectful . . . at first. I told Ruas that I heard he wanted to fight me and I was there to fight him. He said that he wanted to fight, but that he would need four months to prepare. This made me feel that he was more interested in capitalizing on the fight than proving himself, which pissed me off. I was the one who walked into that lion's den ready and willing to fight for nothing but honor! It started to get heated, and my dad stepped between us to calm things down.

When Hélio offered to make a list so I could fight everyone in one day, I angrily told my dad that this was not a street lottery. The situation continued to deteriorate as tempers rose, and I told them to contact us when they were ready to fight. Just as we were leaving, Hugo Duarte, an unknown at the time, who was standing behind Ruas, said, "You can put me at the top of that list!" I could see in Hugo's eyes that he wanted to fight me, that he was serious.

I'd gone to the Luta Livre academy to fight Marco Ruas, an accomplished, reputable fighter, and now I was getting pressured into fighting an upstart. I couldn't challenge a nobody, so I had a friend tell Hugo to meet me at Pepê Beach on Saturday. I got sick the week of the fight and was thinking about postponing it until my messenger called and said, "It's all set! Hugo will be there on Saturday!" Now I knew that there was no backing out, so I started to eat well and get ready.

About forty guys assembled at the Gracie Barra Academy on Saturday morning. I wanted to make sure that this would be a one-on-one fight, so I was giving everyone his instructions. I told my cousin Jean Jacques Machado to watch my back, because I would be surrounded by fighters from both sides. Then my cousin Carlos Gracie Jr. asked me if this fight was worth it. He said, "You have everything to lose and nothing to win!" It's one thing to question my decision weeks or even days before a fight, but it's quite another to do so on the day of the fight, let alone minutes before it.

There were Gracies like my father and brother Rolls, who were always in the front line, and there were others who were not. All the Gracies of our generation learned the martial art and shared the same ideology, but not all became great fighters. Because I fought and beat the Hawaiian and Zulu, I became Rickson Gracie. I was no longer just Hélio Gracie's son. Yes, I had the name, but if I had not fought and won these bouts, that would have been all that I had. I told Carlos that it was better for me to fight Hugo now because if I didn't, no-body else would. "The time for thinking is over, my brother," I told him, "Now it is time to do it." A tense silence fell over the Gracie Barra Academy that was broken by my son, Rock-son, who was only seven. "And if he brings his son, I'm going to kick *his* ass too!" Everybody laughed, which lightened the mood, until someone opened the door and yelled, "The Luta Livre guys are down at Pepê Beach!"

At that time, I had no reservations about bringing my son to this fight. After all, this was our family business, and there were times when a message needed to be sent. We left as a group, and when we got to Pepê Beach, Hugo was there, supported by Eugênio Tadeu and many of the top Luta Livre fighters. We both knew why we were there, so I walked up to Hugo and slapped him in the face. He took off his shirt and sandals, and we began to wrestle on our feet until I was able to drag him to the ground. Hugo used my ponytail to control my head and stood back up. He fell on top on me, then I swept him, but my knee got buried in the sand and Hugo escaped. We stood back up again and smashed into a vendor's stand and went down to the ground again. With the crowd surging all around us, I mounted again, gift-wrapped him, and began to punch him in the face at will. There was nothing he could do to stop the punches.

When I asked Hugo if he wanted to give up, he said, "You'll have to kill me!" so I kept blasting him with punches and elbows. After more blows to the face, he changed his mind, and when he said, "OK, stop!" I let him go.

We stood up and walked to the ocean to wash off the blood and sand. Hugo turned to me and said, "I'm not happy. I was winning until your relatives started kicking me on the ground and throwing sand in my eyes! Typical Gracie bullshit!"

"OK, let's keep fighting then," I replied.

When Hugo said, "No, but we'll meet again!" I knew that this was not over. By the time we got out of the water, Renzo, Royler, and others were skirmishing with Luta Livre fighters. Although the fights got broken up, Royler would fight Eugênio in the coming weeks.

A week later, I was sleeping when my friend pulled up in front of the apartment on his motorcycle and screamed, "Rickson! Those motherfuckers invaded your dad's academy!" I ran down the stairs as fast as I could and jumped on his bike in my underwear. The street that the school was on was filled with people blocking traffic, and the cars and buses were violently honking their horns. We forced our way through the crowd to get to the stairs to the academy, just as my dad, Hugo Duarte, Eugênio Tadeu, and Denilson Maia, the head of the Luta Livre, were coming down. My dad was calm as usual and kept the situation under control.

I saw Hugo and noticed that he was sweaty, already warmed up. We walked over to the concrete patio, where many of the guys with him had T-shirts covering their faces; some had guns, others had knives and broken bottles. These were gangsters, not fighters who lived according to a code. I walked over to Hugo and told him that I wanted to talk to him before we fought. My dad, Hugo, and his teacher, Denilson Maia, went along with me to the backyard.

"Hugo," I said, "I respect the fact that you came here for revenge. I have no problem with that. I'm here to fight you, but this is different than the last fight, because the last time we fought, it was just fighters. Some of these motherfuckers you brought today have no code. Let me tell you one thing: if anyone jumps into this fight before it's over, I will take it very personally."

Hugo said, "No, just you and me."

I nodded and said, "OK, then. Let's do it."

We walked back to the crowd on the patio and squared off. I immediately sensed that Hugo wanted to punch me, so I baited him into throwing a punch. When he did, I deflected it, clinched, and threw him hard onto his back on the concrete. I mounted and started punching him. Hugo covered up to defend his face, but I started banging his head on a stair. He moved his hands to stop me and I punched him in the face. Hugo yelled "Stop! Stop!"

I stopped hitting him and stood up. "You're a tough guy," I said, "You have a bright future as a fighter. Is this matter settled once and for all?"

"Yes," Hugo replied. And I believed him.

Just as we were shaking hands, my younger brother Royler started to fight with Eugenio Tadeu. As we all turned our attention to their fight, a police car pulled up. The cops couldn't get through the crowd, so one of them shot his handgun in the air. Still nobody moved. Then the first cop's partner, a scrawny guy with a thick moustache, blasted his automatic rifle, a bullet from which ricocheted off a building and hit someone in the leg. Finally, Royler and Eugenio stopped fighting, and the crowd scattered. As people tried to get away, the little cop walked to the center of the patio, smiled, and yelled, "Who's the tough guy now?" I thought it funny that the smallest cop was not afraid of anything. It was tragic that it was his gun that put him above the fray. A few days later, Royler and Eugenio fought to a thirty-eight-minute draw.

Looking back today on the fights between Jiu Jitsu and Luta Livre, I see them very differently. At the time, we were all young men full of aggression and testosterone. The rivalry between our two martial arts made all of us better fighters. Steel sharpens steel. We should all be grateful for the fact that we always had the ability to fight one another respectfully. Although there were black eyes, bloody noses, and broken teeth, our fights were always one-on-one and were governed by honor and mutual respect. It was part of the natural competitive process. It was no accident that Marco Ruas, Hugo Duarte, Denilson Maia, Eugenio Tadeu, my brothers, some of my cousins, and I would all go on to fight Mixed Martial Arts professionally in America and Japan.

COMING TO AMERICA

THERE WAS LITTLE LEFT FOR ME TO PROVE IN BRAZIL AT THAT point. America was a bigger stage with more opportunities, and I thought my kids would have a brighter future there. When I decided to move to the US, Kim and I had been separated for over a year and a half. I went to see her and told her that I would like her to come with me and the kids and give our relationship another chance. She agreed to my offer. I wanted to make a fresh start.

I had been to the United States many times but had never lived there. My father told me not to worry about a thing. All I had to do was teach and train, and my brother Rorion would take care of everything else. Problem was, I spoke no English and would be totally dependent on my brother for everything from my green card to a place to live. Initially I was fine with this because I wanted to help him spread the gospel of Gracie Jiu Jitsu to America. Along with Rockson, my mother, and my friend Luis "Limão" (lemon) Heredia, I traveled to the US ahead of Kim and my other children. We moved into Rorion's house in Torrance, a coastal town in Los Angeles County, and taught classes out of his garage. It was an exciting time, and I was totally committed to serving Rorion and the Gracie family.

While I might have been the best fighter in the family, Rorion was by far the best promoter of Gracie Jiu Jitsu. He was a born salesman with a great product to sell, and nothing helped spread Jiu Jitsu more than the portable video camera. After Rorion came to America, he began challenging fighters from other styles and videotaping the bouts. Footage from these and other fights transformed what would have been urban myths into documented truth. In 1988, Rorion put together a video called *Gracie in Action*, which he advertised in the back of martial-arts magazines and sold by mail order. It is important to remember that at that time, there was no internet, much less YouTube. Martial artists traded videotapes like religious artifacts, and none was more valuable than *Gracie in Action*. What Rorion's video lacked in production quality it more than made up for with action. It featured my beach fight with Hugo Duarte, my second bout with Zulu, some of the Luta Livre–versus–Jiu Jitsu matches, and challenge matches with martial artists from various styles in America. Some of my brother's narration was intentionally provocative and meant to challenge other fighting styles. The tape was big and bold, and it was an eye-opener for American fighters in the 1980s, who were mostly strikers and not grapplers. The Gracie challenge had arrived.

For a time, all of my brothers and cousins were successful in our united mission to introduce Gracie Jiu Jitsu to America. Our students regularly fought and won challenge matches against other fighters and then converted them into students—Chuck Norris for one. The actor and American martial-arts icon was not only a great early supporter but was also a dedicated student who eventually earned his black belt. In the 1980s Norris took a vacation to Rio. Everywhere he went, he heard about Gracie Jiu Jitsu and the exploits of my family. Norris contacted my dad and arranged to have a private lesson. After I grappled with him, my dad told Norris to mount him, and when he did, said, "OK, Chuck, punch me." The American hesitated, as my dad was in his seventies by then, but Hélio kept insisting. Finally, Norris drew back his arm to punch, but before he could throw one, the old man had choked him out. Chuck left Brazil impressed by the Gracie family and invited us to come to America and hold a seminar for his students.

So there I was in 1988, arriving in Las Vegas to conduct a seminar for a Hollywood icon. Because Rorion's English was fluent, he served as the master of ceremonies while I and nine of my brothers and cousins taught the students.

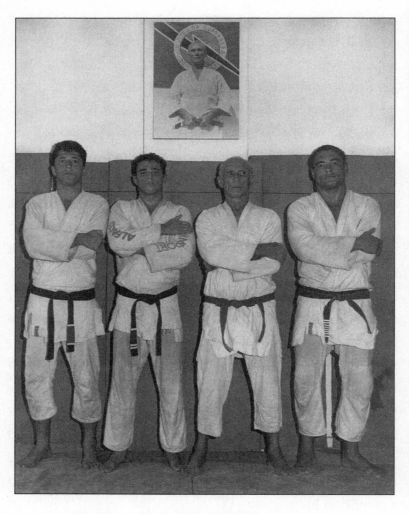

ROLKER, ROYLER, HÉLIO, AND RICKSON GRACIE.
PHOTOGRAPH COURTESY OF BRUCE WEBER.

Chuck Norris rolled out the red carpet for us in Las Vegas and gave us an extremely respectful introduction. After Rorion read a letter from Hélio congratulating Norris for having the wisdom to invite us, Rorion and I demonstrated some self-defense moves. Then I had a friendly match with Chuck. I let him close the distance and throw a kick, but I got him in clinch, took him down, and had him in a choke in about a minute. Even though the seminar was a great success, afterward, Rorion and the actor had a disagreement over money. Not only did Rorion lose him as a student, but Chuck Norris hired our cousins the Machado brothers (Carlos, Rigan, Roger, Jean Jacques, and John), to teach him.

The Machados came from a more stable upper-middle-class background than we did. Their father was a judge and they did not grow up in Rio. Not only were they much more reasonable than Rorion, they were great Jiu Jitsu fighters and teachers in their own right. My cousin Jean Jacques Machado is an inspiring person who went on to become one of the greatest Jiu Jitsu teachers in America. Born with only a thumb and part of a pinkie on one of his hands, Jean Jacques learned how to adapt and improvise better than anyone I had ever seen. His Jiu Jitsu is both intensely personal and creative.

I got to know Jean Jacques well when he was a teenager and began to travel to Rio to train with me. The seriousness with which he took his training impressed me. If I taught my first lesson at 7:00 a.m., he would be sitting on the curb waiting for me to open the academy when I arrived. He would spend the whole morning watching me teach, smartly observing until it was time to train. And when that time came, he followed all of the Gracie protocols; he had desire, willpower, athletic ability, and humility. Even as a purple belt, Jean Jacques was giving the black belts a hard time on the mat. He would go on to become one of the Gracie family's greatest Jiu Jitsu and grappling competitors.

Chuck Norris was so impressed by the Machados that he gave them a school of their own in a building he owned. Even worse, word quickly spread that you could learn Gracie Jiu Jitsu from them without having to deal with Rorion. The Machados received a great deal of support from prominent American martial artists like wrestler Gene LeBell and many others. They would not be the only Gracies to challenge my brother's authority and go their own way once they arrived in America. The Gracie clan was splitting and factionalizing in the States, and there was nothing that my brother could do about it. Just like our Scottish ancestors, Gracie clan leaders were beginning to feud.

In addition to a black belt, Rorion also had a law degree, which he often used to press his advantage and overplay his hand with in business dealings. This left many family members with bitter feelings. Even though Hélio wanted Rorion to lead the Gracies in America, it was easier said than done. There were just too many of us moving in different directions, and Rorion's efforts to control the clan backfired. After he threatened to sue members of the Gracie family, whom he had grown up on the mats with, for using their own—

Gracie—last name, many family members surrendered. Gracie Jiu Jitsu got renamed "Brazilian Jiu Jitsu." I believe that if my brother had allowed everyone to use our family name, our martial art would still be called Gracie Jiu Jitsu today, and perhaps it'd be even bigger than it is.

Even worse for Rorion, bloodied and charismatic Gracie warriors like my cousin Renzo would soon come to America, posing yet another threat to his monopoly. I had known Renzo and his two brothers, Ralph and Ryan, since they were boys. After their father and mother, Robson and Vera, divorced, Renzo became a father figure to his younger brothers Ralph and Ryan and to many others. By the time he arrived in America, he was already leading many of the younger Gracies and other friends who lacked direction. Renzo was a born fighter who, rather than getting scared in dangerous situations, got focused.

Renzo would go on to be one of the most successful Jiu Jitsu teachers. I once asked a student who trained with both of us what his academy in New York City was like, and he said, "It's a tough school. Imagine if you took ten babies and threw them into the deep end of a swimming pool. Nine of them would probably drown, but the survivor will become an Olympic swimmer. For white belts, that's kind of what Renzo's academy is like." In addition to being a fearless MMA fighter, Renzo has a big heart, which I believe has contributed to his success. Because Renzo experienced the beneficial aspects of all our family members training together, he re-created this atmosphere in New

York City and encouraged many of the younger Gracies to move to America. Once they arrived in the States, he gave them jobs, places to stay, and took them all under his wing. What I like most about Renzo is that the better he did, the more generous he became.

Unlike Renzo and the Machados, I initially did not have the option of breaking away from Rorion. Because I got my green card through my brother, I couldn't receive money under my name or even open a bank account. When Kim and my other three kids arrived in America, the pressure on me increased dramatically. In addition to teaching at Rorion's academy, I also taught classes at a health club in Laguna Beach. I was supposed to give my brother all of the money I made teaching, and he was supposed to pay all of my expenses. But as my following grew larger and the checks got bigger, I was not seeing any more money. Our relationship hit a new low when he told me that he might take away my green card if I didn't follow his orders.

Working for my brother was becoming more and more unpleasant, so I decided to take a leap of faith and open my own academy. Kim had brought her savings, so we had a little bit of a nest egg that we used to gain our independence. When my brother lost control of me, I became his greatest adversary, because I had the image, ability, and leadership skills that he lacked, and worst of all, everyone knew it.

The West LA Karate School rented me their school on Pico Boulevard in an industrial section of Los Angeles. It was a traditional Japanese karate school, complete with a raised wooden platform, *makiwara* striking post, and an oil painting of an old Japanese karate master. Hot in the summer and cold in the winter, my school had no sign, no parking, no windows, no showers, and it was almost impossible to find. But since I was the family champion and California was buzzing about Gracie Jiu Jitsu, it did not take long for dangerous men from all over the world to find this rundown karate dojo tucked away in an alley next to an auto-body shop.

Most of my first generation of students were aspiring professional fighters, lifelong martial artists from other styles, surfers, or professional men of action who used physical force in their daily occupations: soldiers, cops, prison guards, and bouncers. That's what I mean by dangerous. Some wanted to learn while others just wanted to test their skills against us, but in the end almost all of them became dedicated Gracie Jiu Jitsu students.

My Pico Academy was a neutral environment where you had to leave your preconceptions and prejudices in the locker room. I didn't allow them onto my mats.

I was spreading my family's art and meeting interesting people, and many became lifelong friends who enriched my life and opened my mind to things that I had never experienced.

Jiu Jitsu students choose to step into an environment where the natural constants are turmoil, confusion, fear, and aggression. Jiu Jitsu can bring together people who have natural antagonisms toward one another. It was hard and sometimes awkward when a pot grower rolled with a cop, but there was no better place for them to connect, because a Jiu Jitsu academy is the most neutral place they will ever meet. They think they don't like each other, but then they develop mutual respect after training together week after week.

Some teachers are only concerned with making fighters and have no regard for the other positive aspects of martial arts. My schools were never like that. I enjoyed taking guys with small bodies but big hearts and minds—Pedro Sauer, Luis "Limão" Heredia, my brother Royler—and turning them into champions. I was never impressed by someone's size or physique. I learned to judge people by their humility and their self-respect.

I loved teaching Jiu Jitsu because it revealed a person's true personality. When I stepped onto the mat I saw people dressed in white, and they all had belts around their waists. Once they engaged, it was impossible to hide their nerves and their fear. Sometimes a small, soft-looking guy was the true warrior because he was resilient and brave in both victory and defeat. The coward was fine when he was kicking ass, but as soon as he got in a bad position, he would be the first to exclaim, "Stop! I'm hurt! Stop! I'm tired! Stop! I'm old!" It was easy to read the mind of a coward, even if they are naturally aggressive.

I tried to get my students to examine not just how they fought, but also how they felt when they fought. If they did so honestly, I could help them rebuild themselves as stronger people. However, growth only came if they were willing to face their shortcomings with pride, and only if they did their homework. But anyone who was willing to come into my gym and continue to come back would know better than to not do their homework.

The invisible aspects of Jiu Jitsu like the sense of touch, weight, momentum, and physical connection to your opponent are very difficult to teach. This is not rational, intellectual knowledge that one can learn from a lecture or a book—only thousands of hours of training—and some of my American students were getting it in record time.

The Pico Academy wasn't all fun and games, however. Every school needs a clear leader who is the students' point of reference, because a Jiu Jitsu academy is like a circus, and it takes on the personality of its ringmaster. In every school there are tigers, lions, bears, snakes, dogs, cats . . . even lizards. After the ringmaster tames the lions, he must keep them from eating the dogs, and then he must keep the dogs from eating the cats, and the cats from eating the lizards, and so on. Because I led by example, I had to crack the hard nuts the minute they walked through my door. If I didn't tame the monsters on day one, they would return to my school to feast on white belts like raw meat.

Whenever an intimidating guy, like 250-pound Greco-Roman wrestler and early MMA fighter Stefanos Miltsakakis, came to the Pico Academy, I dealt with him directly. Stefanos had been a heavyweight on the Greek national wrestling team, had kickboxed, and was an especially good grappler on his feet. A mutual friend brought him to the academy, and

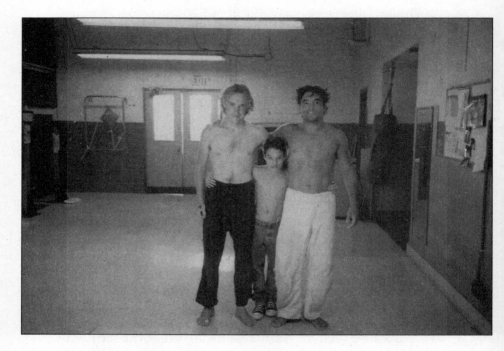

PETER MAGUIRE, ROCKSON GRACIE, RICKSON GRACIE, PICO ACADEMY.
PHOTOGRAPH COURTESY OF THE RICKSON GRACIE COLLECTION.

Stefanos asked respectfully if we could train. When someone says, "Let's train," it can mean anything from a friendly grappling match to an all-out brawl. When the big Greek came out of the locker room wearing only Muay Thai shorts, I asked him what rules he wanted. I suggested *vale tudo*, but he was taken aback and said, "I only wanted to grapple." In those days, I always let first-time visitors know that I was willing to go as far as they wanted to take it.

We engaged on our feet and pushed and pulled for close to ten minutes. When we finally went to the ground, Stefanos put his knee on my face and showed me that he understood the importance of discomfort in a fight. I knew that the pace was unsustainable for him, and after he exhausted himself, I took his back and submitted him with a choke. In twenty-five minutes of hard grappling, I made him tap five or six more times. He was shocked and disappointed afterward. "Nobody's ever done that to me!" he said, before asking if he could be my student. I was happy to have Stefanos as both a student and a sentry at the Pico Academy. Not only did he raise the level of performance, but he also served as one of the school's bouncers when necessary.

I could not be at the academy all the time and needed frontline soldiers to regulate things in my absence. In addition to the formal and informal Gracie challenges to be fought, my stronger students had to protect my weaker ones. For example, a big kickboxer whom nobody knew once showed up at the morning class. During a simple takedown drill, he kneed a white belt half his size in the face and broke his nose. Not only was this move unnecessary, it was obvious to everyone watching that it was not an accident. Luis "Limão" sent the white belt to the bathroom to stanch his bleeding and spoke in Portuguese to the Brazilian students, who translated his simple message for their American classmates: "We don't want this asshole in here. He crossed the line by beating up on a white belt, and now he must pay." For the next forty minutes, the kickboxer was thrown, submitted, and stretched over and over. He never again returned to Pico Academy.

It was also important for my students to see and know that nobody, including me, was above the fray. I never asked my students to do anything that I was not prepared to do myself. If you stepped onto my mats, I was going to push you the same way I pushed myself. Sometimes I chose to surprise my students. After surfing, I liked to show up at the morning class just before the hard rolling was about to begin. Even Limão would stiffen up when I walked in unannounced. I liked to shock everyone to their senses by putting them in unbearable situations that would force them to deal with the kind of fear that's normal in a fight and teach them how to manage it. As Gracies, we were taught that there was no shame in being nervous or afraid; what mattered was what you did in the face of fear. The more I knew about my students' strengths and weaknesses, the more I could teach them. It was better to learn these hard and sometimes humbling lessons behind closed doors, among friends, than out on the street.

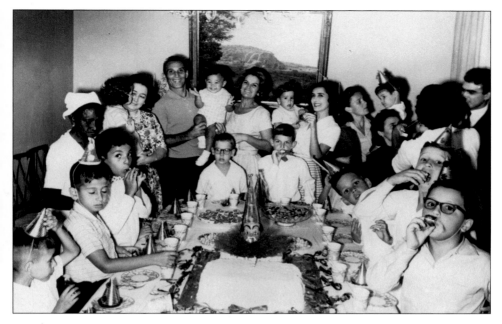

HÉLIO, RICKSON, AND
MARGARIDA GRACIE AT
RICKSON'S SECOND
BIRTHDAY PARTY.
*PHOTOGRAPH COURTESY OF THE
RICKSON GRACIE COLLECTION.*

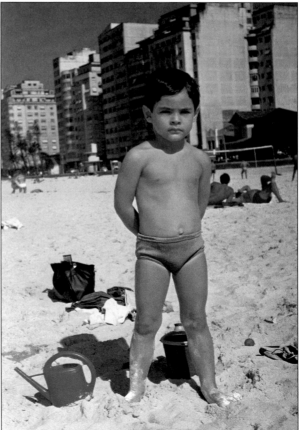

RICKSON GRACIE AT
COPACABANA BEACH.
*PHOTOGRAPH COURTESY OF THE
RICKSON GRACIE COLLECTION.*

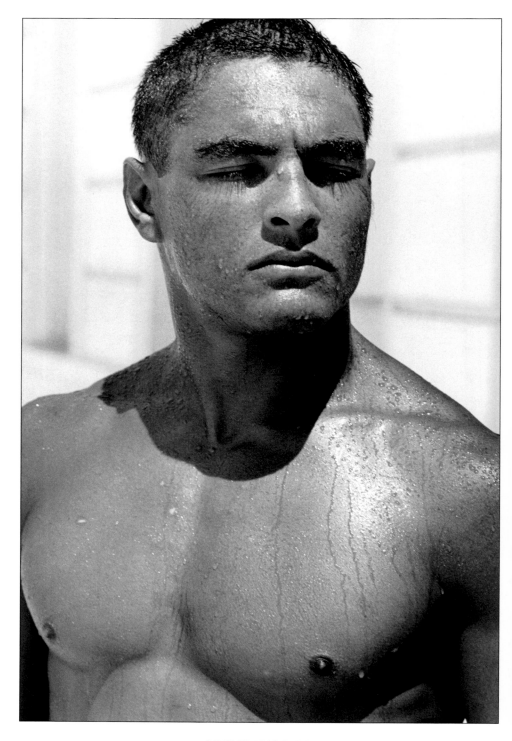

RICKSON GRACIE, RIO.
PHOTOGRAPH COURTESY OF BRUCE WEBER.

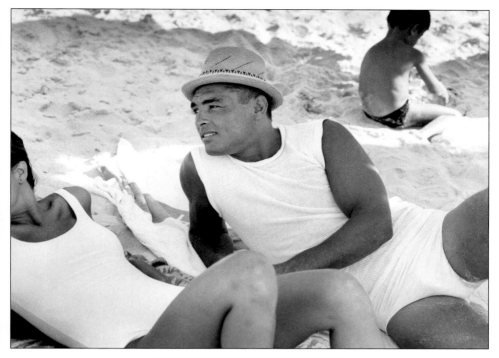

RICKSON AND KIM GRACIE, COPACABANA.
PHOTOGRAPH COURTESY OF BRUCE WEBER.

RICKSON GRACIE, RIO DE JANEIRO, 1988.
PHOTOGRAPH COURTESY OF MARCOS PRADO / @REVISTATRIP, 1988.

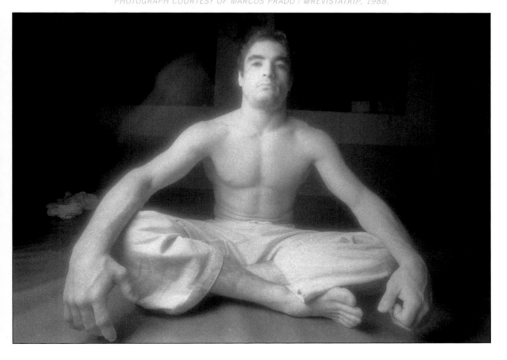

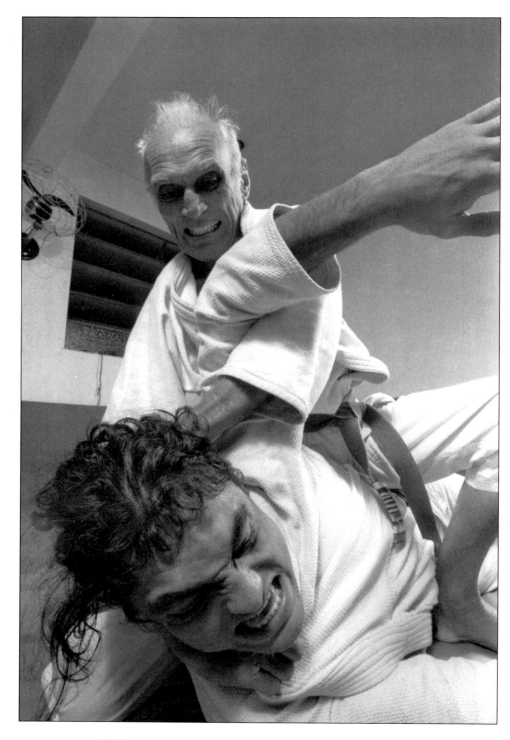

HÉLIO AND RICKSON GRACIE TRAINING IN RIO DE JANEIRO, 1988.
PHOTOGRAPH COURTESY OF MARCOS PRADO / @REVISTATRIP, 1988.

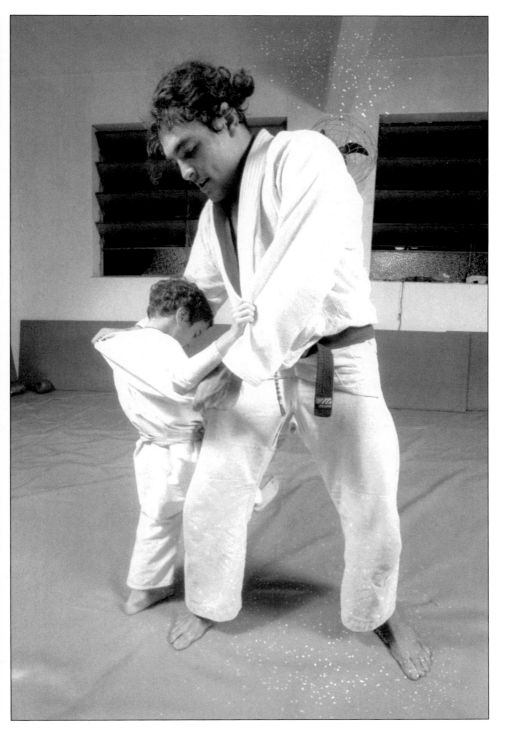

RICKSON AND ROCKSON GRACIE, 1988.
PHOTOGRAPH COURTESY OF MARCOS PRADO / @REVISTATRIP, 1988.

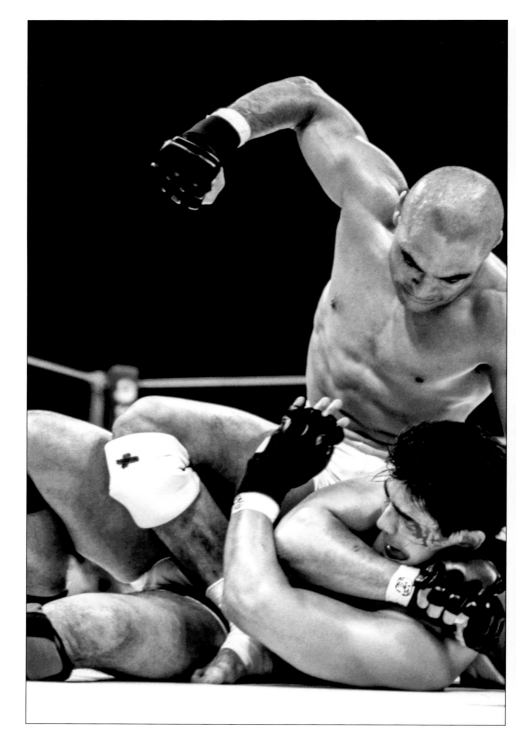

RICKSON GRACIE PUNCHES MASAKATSU FUNAKI, 2000.
PHOTOGRAPH COURTESY OF SUSUMU NAGAO.

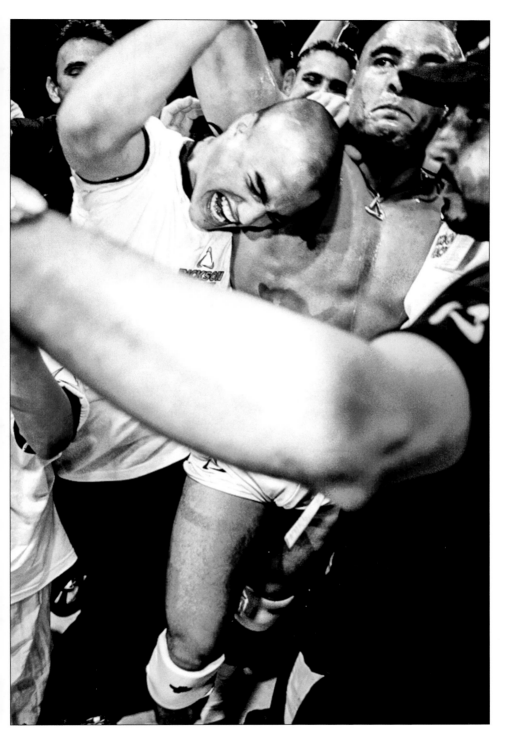

ROCKSON AND RICKSON GRACIE AFTER THE MASAKATSU FUNAKI FIGHT, 2000.
PHOTOGRAPH COURTESY OF SUSUMU NAGAO.

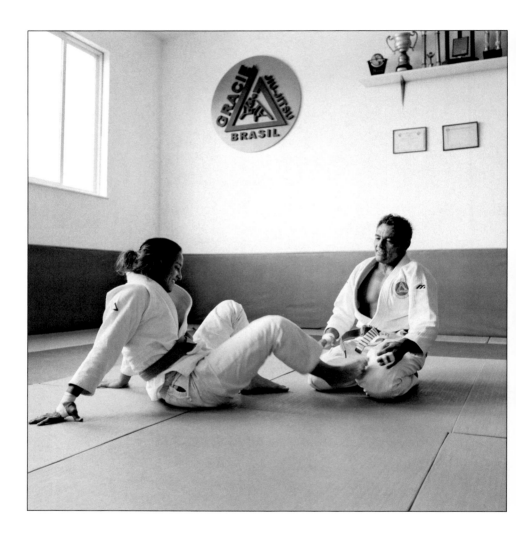

RICKSON AND KAULIN GRACIE, 2014.
PHOTOGRAPH COURTESY OF STEFAN KOCEV.

Some days I would tell the students to line up against the wall and then announce that I was going to have a grappling match, starting on the feet, with every single person there. Other days, I would have an expert striker put on boxing gloves and make my students try to take him down without getting punched. This drill taught students which ranges of distance are dangerous and which are safe. And this is essential because it taught the advantage and disadvantages of fighting a person on the ground versus fighting them on their feet. They learned how to close the distance and safely take the fight to the ground. After all, you can't fight on the ground if you can't take your opponent down.

Surprise in-house tournaments were another favorite of mine. These tournaments had no trophies, spectators, points, or traditional time limits. The only judge was the jury of your peers. I would whistle and say, "Everyone up against the wall," at which point the room would get very quiet. When I said, "160 pounds and below to my left, 160 and above to my right," you could hear a pin drop. These competitions allowed me to shatter the factions, cliques, and egos that are so common in martial arts schools. Instead, I built a clear and honest hierarchy whereby everyone knew his place in my academy's food chain. Some guys would beat everyone during informal training sessions but choke in competition. Others rose to the occasion and surprised themselves. A student might be a king one day for a day, but with success came new, higher expectations from me.

During one of our in-house tournaments, I pitted one of

my scrawniest white belts against a formidable college water polo player. During his first interclass tournament, the white belt got caught in an armlock, refused to tap out, and got his elbow capsule popped. Still, he came to class the next day. When the match started, the water polo player took him down and walked right into a triangle choke. Without saying a word, my Brazilian students, using pantomime gestures, silently coached the white belt who followed their directions and got the water polo player in a triangle choke. After the bout, I could tell by the look on my white belt's face that he was more surprised than anyone else. Rather than treat this win as a fluke, it filled him with confidence. He improved quickly, and his newfound confidence bled over into other parts of his life. Soon he was attaining professional goals that he had once never thought possible.

While some people are impressive natural athletes, some have a never-say-die attitude that cannot be taught. The latter often go further in Jiu Jitsu and in life. It didn't matter to me if a student won easily or lost badly. I never focused on who won. I tried to inspire the losers as much as the winners. If a student won, I would simply say, "Props to you for winning, but you could have won smarter and faster. Anyway, congrats." If he lost, the lesson was, "Congrats, you could have made worse mistakes, and you didn't panic like last time. If you improve your armlock defense, you won't lose to him again." I respected every one of my students for just stepping onto the mat and measuring himself against another man.

Orlando Cani made me realize that anyone could teach you something, especially your students. Sure, I could beat them in Jiu Jitsu, but over the years I've had students who were great musicians or brilliant scholars, and all of them taught me things I would have never learned had I put myself on a pedestal. I realized at a very early age the value of interacting with people from all walks of life. I was always curious and interested in anyone who did something really well. Fishing, bull riding, painting, singing, art—it didn't matter—I have always admired ability in all of its manifestations. I was never jealous or envious; in fact, sometimes I wish I could've spent more time learning different things.

When we first came to the US, Kim and I were working our asses off just to get by. While life on the mat was always the same, life off the mat was more difficult, because America was so different from Brazil. Like the United States, Brazil had been a colony, but it was one where Europeans at first went primarily to fill their boats with gold and emeralds, fuck some beautiful brown women, and go home. In contrast, America had a much more idealistic Constitution and grew into a more orderly society—literally. People here did things that I had never seen before: they stood in line, stopped for traffic lights, and mostly obeyed the laws. These may seem like obvious requirements for a workable society, but to me this was a strange new world. My transition to living in American society was not always smooth.

My first wake-up call about how different life was in the US came when I bought my first car and began driving. At first, I drove as if I was still in Rio. I ran red lights, drove alone in the carpool lane, and made U-turns whenever and wherever I felt like it. If I hit traffic, I'd pull onto the shoulder and zoom on by. I was no sheep and was sure that I could outsmart everyone, but I soon learned otherwise. One day I was going surfing with some friends, and we didn't have proper racks for the boards, so we just used straps to secure the four surfboards to the roof of the car. It was windy and raining when we got on the freeway, and suddenly we heard an unfamiliar sound. The boards blew off our roof and smashed into the windshield of the car behind us.

We stopped to pick up the boards. The driver of the car the boards hit was so pissed off that he crossed the freeway and drove back to us! It turned out that he was an off-duty California Highway Patrol officer, and he demanded to know who was driving. I told him that I was the driver and handed him my paperwork. I told him that my insurance would pay for the damage to his car, and I almost had him calmed down. Then Coyote, a Brazilian friend and student who had dreadlocks and was covered in tattoos, approached, put his hand on the cop's shoulder, and said, "Hey, officer, no problem."

The cop jumped back and barked, "Take your hands off me!" Although I was able to resolve that situation without getting arrested or shot, I kept getting ticket after ticket and soon lost my driver's license. The lesson? Problems could not be "fixed" in Los Angeles the same way they could be in Rio.

In Brazil, there are many ways to resolve a problem. In America, however, you are held accountable to the law most of the time. Most people in the US obey the rules because the laws themselves are rigid; there isn't much room to get around them. If an American gets arrested for stealing a bike when he is eighteen, his life can be defined by this one stupid decision. In Brazil, whatever you do before the age of twenty-one is largely forgotten. Because we can't rely on the law, Brazilians learn to improvise and must play the right cards at the right time. There are many more jokers and wild cards in the Brazilian deck than the American one.

Waiting in line was also a new experience. I had never stood in a line in my life, because in Brazil you force your way to the front. Everyone does. Not in America. One day, I went to the pharmacy to buy something and the shop-keeper was talking with an old lady. I tried to interrupt with a quick question, but when I said, "Excuse me, where are the . . ." the shopkeeper looked at me sternly and cut me off. "You will need to excuse me for a moment, sir. I will get to you as soon as I finish with her," he told me. Then he kept talking to the old lady about the hair dye. When it was my turn, the shopkeeper answered all my questions and gave me his full attention. Over time, I began to see the value of obeying these formalities. It was I who had to adjust, not other people.

America was also a much better place for my girls, Kauan and Kaulin, because they could be anything they wanted to be. The girls in the Gracie family never got the same amount of attention as the boys and were not urged to reach for the stars the same way we were. If my dad had had his way, all of the girls would have been wives and mothers and nothing else. I wanted much more for my girls, as did Kim, who was a very dynamic, progressive woman. We both wanted our girls to go far, in whatever directions they chose.

I often had to adopt completely different strategies to teach my children the same lessons because their personalities were so different. Yes, I was their friend, but more important, I was their father, and in order to be a good father, I had to set limits, chart their growth, and have the patience and sensitivity to connect with them. One time I bought the kids their favorite Brazilian guarana drinks. Rockson hid his in the back of the refrigerator so he could drink it after dinner. Kaulin watched him hide it, then went into the kitchen, drank his soda, placed the cap back on the empty bottle, and put it back in the refrigerator. After dinner, Rockson went to get his soda, discovered it was empty, and came to me and said, "Kaulin drank my soda." Kaulin just sat there looking totally innocent as though she had no idea what he was talking about. So I turned to Kaulin and said, "Don't lie to Papa. Tell me the truth now. It will be better for you than if you lie."

"OK, I did it," she said, confessing only because I was the person asking. If Rockson had asked her, she would have denied it, yelled back at him, and fought him, if necessary. I preferred honesty rather than strict punishment, openness rather than condemnation.

Moving was probably hardest for Rockson. In a few short months, he had gone from being the prince of Rio to just another skinny Hispanic-looking kid in a California public school who didn't speak English. And his being physically small compared to most of the American kids made him insecure. All the ESL classes in the world can't help that. One morning he came out of his room to go to school with football shoulder pads on under his shirt and insisted on wearing them to school. I said no, of course, but I saw right into the source of his pain.

In an effort to become a leader, Rockson tried to over-compensate with aggression and became extremely reckless in order to prove himself. He would accept any challenge and fight anyone. When I sent him to elementary school in Torrance, he wanted to fight every kid there. At least once a month, the principal would call me screaming: "Rockson fought six kids today! He doesn't understand the rules of basketball and won't let the other kids have the ball." Another time, Rockson came home with a backpack full of candy. He told me some bullshit story about how he'd "found" it, but I knew that he'd stolen it. Even my punishing him did little to correct his behavior. I have been a fighter my entire life, so I understand putting myself at risk, but the ways Rockson was putting himself at risk were not rational or intelligent.

This trait had always been with him. When he was very young, Rockson once said to his sister, "I'm either going to be rich, in prison, or dead." Can you imagine a kid saying that? He was drawn like a magnet to trouble that he easily could have avoided. This imbalance concerned me, because it took Rockson out of a zone of comfort and put him constantly on the edge. I was not just watching another aggressive Gracie growing up; I was watching someone with an unbalanced mental approach to life. When Kim tried to rein him in, he became rebellious and defiant toward her. This caused strife between Kim and me because she did not want her kids to be Gracie brawlers. She'd hoped that the move to America would put them on a different track, but it was too late: Rockson was already on a self-guided mission to be the greatest Gracie of his generation—reckless, yes, but forever a fighter.

By 1992, my academy was thriving, my students were dramatically improving, and nobody was picking up Jiu Jitsu faster than the wrestlers, who had come in droves. It was hard for them to get used to fighting off of their backs, but they understood the ground and had amazing work ethics. When I went to Utah to teach a seminar at my old friend Pedro Sauer's academy, I was introduced to Olympic wrestling gold medalist Mark Schultz, who was coaching in Utah at the time. Schultz was gracious and friendly, and I was impressed that he even wanted to train with me. What did America's greatest wrestler have to gain by rolling with me? He was brave simply for having a mind open enough to risk himself in a new martial art.

Once the niceties were over, I asked Schultz if he wanted *vale tudo* rules, but he said he just wanted to grapple. Once we began, I knew that there was no way I was going to tackle Mark Schultz, so I pulled him into my guard and got him in a triangle choke with my legs. *That was quick!* I thought. He was mad when he tapped because he hadn't seen it coming and still didn't understand what I'd done. To get choked by the legs of a man on his back was eye-opening for a wrestler at that time.

True student of the sport that he was, Schultz was much more cautious in our next match. He stayed on top of me while I let him use every tool in his toolbox. Schultz eventually got me in a cradle hold and cranked my neck. It was uncomfortable, but I knew that wrestlers couldn't maintain this explosive pace for long because their usual matches are only five minutes long. He didn't know how to perform submissions yet, and I was never going to tap just from pressure. It took me about ten minutes to cook him down. Once he started to get tired, I took his back and submitted him with a choke.

A two-time world champion and Olympic gold medalist is not used to losing, and Mark Schultz was *upset*, even more so than the first time. I told him that he was a great champion and that if we had been wrestling, the outcome would have been different because I would have been playing by his rules rather than mine. He nodded and said he understood. In the end, Schultz fell in love with Jiu Jitsu, trained with Pedro Sauer, earned his black belt, fought in the UFC, and became a great representative of our martial art. Mark Schultz was an honest and humble man for whom I'll always have respect.

In early 1993, Rorion's dream of bringing *vale tudo* fighting to America to showcase Jiu Jitsu was about to come true.

He asked me to meet with him and his student, Hollywood director John Milius, and told me that they had backers for the Ultimate Fighting Championship, America's first *vale tudo* event. Finally, an opportunity for me to make a name for myself fighting in America! This was the opportunity that I had moved to the United States for, and now it was a reality.

When Rorion told me that he wanted our younger brother Royce to fight in the first tournament and keep me as backup in case he lost, I was disappointed. While this seemed like a sensible decision, there were other reasons for it. Because Rorion and I were not getting along at the time of the first UFC, he didn't want to risk making me a star who would overshadow him. My younger brother Royce was a happy-go-lucky kid who had never won a significant Jiu Jitsu title, much less a *vale tudo* match. He was, however, the most manageable Gracie and, for a time, Rorion had the same, almost paternal, relationship with him that my father had had with my uncle Carlos.

Nevertheless, I liked Royce and wanted him to do well. I agreed to train him for his first fight for a small percentage of the $50,000 purse if he won. During the summer of 1993, Royce and I would meet at the Pico Academy. He was no match for me, so I was able to push him to his breaking point and then beyond it. When I sensed that he had had enough, I would kiss his cheek, pat him on the head, and call it a day. As the date of the first UFC approached, I felt confident that if Royce stuck to the Gracie game plan of avoiding punches and taking the fight to the ground, he could win. During the week prior to the fight, I started to get his mind ready. I told him that winning was OK, losing was OK, and dying was OK. He should be happy to be in America representing the family.

The first Ultimate Fighting Championship was a single elimination tournament held in the McNichols Sports Arena in Denver, Colorado, in November of 1993. It was much closer to *vale tudo* than today's MMA. There were no gloves, no weight divisions, no rounds, and no time limits. I did not like the way that Rorion's partners had promoted the event as a human cockfight. All of their television and print ads announced that "there are no rules," which was not entirely true. It was too sensational. Yes, bare-knuckle fighting can be bloody, but it is nowhere near as harmful to the brain as boxing or today's MMA. Boxers and current MMA fighters suffer much more brain trauma because they wear gloves and have taped hands. Without them, fighters would break their hands hitting someone in the head over and over, thus mitigating the potential for repeat blows.

My dad and I, along with Relson, Royler, and a big contingent of Gracies, students, and friends, traveled to Colorado to support Royce in his first fight. Once we got there, I took Royce aside and told him that I did not want to see him laughing or joking until the tournament was over. He needed to be calm and focused, I explained, because when he walked into the cage he would be all alone.

Up until the rules meeting the day before the fight, Royce was managing his nerves pretty well. At 175 pounds, he was by far the smallest and least experienced of the eight fighters in the event. The other seven men were all over six feet tall and over 200 pounds; Teila Tuli, the Samoan Sumo wrestler, weighed 420 pounds.

As I explained, the first UFC was billed as a competition with no rules, but there were actually three: no biting, eye gouging, or groin strikes. As soon as the rules meeting began, the fighters started to argue. One of the big kickboxers wanted to be able to throw groin strikes and wouldn't stop trading words with Rorion. When he accused my brother of rigging the tournament for Royce to win, the situation got heated. Fighters and their camps stood up and shouted insults. The tension increased until Tuli, the Sumo wrestler, said, "I just signed my paper. I don't know about you guys, but I came here to party. If anyone else came here to party, I'll see you tomorrow night at the arena." Then the big Samoan put his signed paper down on the table and walked out. Rorion eventually put this coup down, but it did little to settle Royce's nerves less than twenty-four hours before his first *vale tudo* fight.

After we got to the arena on fight night, I could sense that Royce's case of nerves had gotten worse. And Rorion's own fear was palpable, because he had spent years putting this showcase for Gracie Jiu Jitsu together, but now he had to consider the possibility that his decision to put Royce in the tournament might backfire. I walked over to Royce and quietly held him in an attempt to calm him down. I told him that I knew exactly what he was experiencing because I felt the same way during my first fight with Zulu. "You will do fine. You are prepared, and I will be there for you every step of the way," I said. "Now, breathe. Let's get ready, it will all be over soon. The hard work is over, Royce. None of these guys will be worse than training with me." That was true. Although he didn't know it, I did for Royce exactly what Rolls had done for me many years ago in Brasília.

From the dressing room we could hear the bloodthirsty crowd roar when the Samoan Sumo wrestler got his teeth kicked out (as we found out later). A few minutes later, a UFC official poked his head in the door and told us to get ready to make our way to the ring. Royce got to his feet with a look of nervous determination. I had steadied him for his all-important first fight, with boxer Art Jimmerson. Royler, Relson, and I led him to the ring, and as we approached it, my father rushed out of the crowd and ran next to me shouting instructions into my ear. Once a general, always a general.

After Royce beat the boxer without getting hit and then made Ken Shamrock, the fighter who posed the biggest threat to him, tap in less than a minute, his confidence resurfaced. In the final, Royce faced a tall, dead-eyed Dutch kickboxer named Gerard Gordeau and stuck with the same winning formula. When Royce took him down to the ground and was just about to choke him, Gordeau bit Royce's ear. After he freed his ear, Royce choked him, and when he tapped, Royce kept choking him and did not stop until the referee pried him off Gordeau.

The UFC had forced Royce to unleash a new ferocity.

Normally easygoing and unassuming, Royce summoned a deep strength, and I was proud of him for answering this challenge. Today, many criticize the first UFC as an infomercial for Gracie Jiu Jitsu, but it is important to remember that in order for Royce to win that first tournament, he still had to defeat three much larger opponents in a single night. This is no small feat for any fighter. After Royce won the tournament in less than five minutes of total fighting time, Americans were stunned and amazed by the power and efficiency of Gracie Jiu Jitsu. Overnight, Royce Gracie became the biggest name in martial arts, and Gracie Jiu Jitsu exploded in popularity.

Rorion thought it was hard to control Gracies, but soon America would be flooded with non–family members who represented the good, the bad, and the ugly of my family's martial art. During the 1990s, an unusual thing happened to Brazilians when they flew to the US. Some of their belts magically turned from blue to brown, and even worse, from purple to black. In the land of the blind, the one-eyed man is king.

THE LAND OF
THE RISING SUN

AFTER THE UFC PROMOTERS HAD OVERSOLD THE FIRST EVENT
as a human cockfight, they attracted a pro wrestling audience that was completely ignorant about real fighting. For
example, every time a fight went to the ground at the first
UFC, the spectators booed because they didn't understand
what they were watching. They wanted a barroom brawl.
Rather than educate and uplift the fans, the UFC built its
rules around their whims by breaking fights into short
rounds and making fighters stand up who would normally
fight on the ground. Today, 98 percent of MMA fans have
never stepped into the cage, or even onto the mat, much

less felt their noses break or tendons pop. Their relationship with violence is virtual. MMA is just something else to watch on a screen. Perhaps this is why the UFC's Octagon is now the equivalent of the Roman Colosseum. Bloody, violent, and explosive. Still, one interesting thing did happen for me after UFC 2. When I appeared with Royce in his post-fight interview, he thanked me and acknowledged that I was ten times better than him. People suddenly got interested in me—especially the Japanese.

I had always wanted to fight in Japan because of its martial arts history and culture. Unlike the Americans, they understood fighting. My student and early MMA fighter Erik Paulson introduced me to retired Japanese pro wrestler Yori Nakamura, who worked for the Shooto Association, one of Japan's earliest MMA organizations. Long before the UFC, Shooto had gloves, rounds, weight divisions, and a sophisticated audience. Unlike American MMA audiences, who have been raised on Jackie Chan movies and pro wrestling, when fights went to the ground, the Japanese audiences would quietly "Ohhh" and "Ahhh" like a tennis crowd. There was nowhere else on Earth where fighters were held in such high esteem.

The Japanese promoters invited me to fight in one of their tournaments, but when they offered me only $3,000, I felt disrespected and said no. Then my wife, Kim, stepped into the negotiations. She told them that if they wanted me to fight, it would be under *vale tudo* rules, and it would be for *much more* money. In the end, Kim's patience and persistence paid off. She got the Japanese promoters to pay me $50,000 to fight and another $50,000 if I won. That was a lot of money in those days. I would double my price after every win. With Kim acting as my manager, I could now focus only on training for my first *vale tudo* fight in Japan.

When I told Rorion that I planned to fight in Japan, he strongly objected and convinced my dad that I shouldn't fight there. Most of the time, Kim got along with my dad, because he loved our kids and respected her as a mother. But when it came to business and her management of my career, he viewed her as the opposition, because I was supposed to follow Rorion. Kim didn't trust my brother and took me out of his control when she began managing me. My father resented our independence and success, the same way he resented Carlson for opening his own academy in the 1960s. In his mind, if we were going to be successful, it had to be under his wing. But Rorion's plan was already falling apart. More and more Brazilians were coming to the US to fight MMA and open Jiu Jitsu schools. Ironically, Rorion was now a victim of his own success.

My father lived in Brazil and was completely out of touch with what was going on in America. He had no idea how anarchic the world of Jiu Jitsu had gotten in the States. When I asked Hélio to come to Japan to corner me, he declined. This broke my heart, but I still had to fulfill my mission. I now felt like a ronin (a masterless samurai), except that I was not going to commit seppuku or become a mercenary by fighting fixed fights for lots of money. I was now more determined than ever to prove to the world that I was the greatest Gracie.

When I asked Royce if he would come to Japan to corner me, as I had done for him at the first two UFCs, he said that he would like to, but Rorion wouldn't let him. I told Royce that I understood but that I could no longer train him, because I needed to prepare for my upcoming fights in Japan. In the end, the only one of my brothers who rejected Rorion's decree that no Gracie should go to Japan to help me was my younger brother Royler. He told Rorion, "You are my brother, I love you and will always be there to support Royce, but you are not going to forbid me from helping Rickson. He is also my brother. He did a lot for me, and I am not going to turn my back on him now." I was grateful to have Royler in my training camp and in my corner. In the coming years, he would become one of my most important supporters.

A month before my first fight in Japan, Royce fought in UFC 3 without me in his corner. I watched the event on television, and when I saw Kimo, his massive, steroid-swollen opponent, walk to the ring with a wooden cross the size of a telephone pole on his back, I sensed trouble. Kimo easily defended Royce's takedowns and landed some big punches. Royce finally managed to get him on the ground, but Kimo took his back and began to punch him. My brother weathered more heavy blows before he was able to grab Kimo's ponytail, control his head, and secure an armlock. Royce won the bout but had to be carried out of the ring and could not answer the bell for his next fight. Needless to say, UFC 3 would not be won by a Gracie.

By pitting "villain" characters, like Kimo and Tank Abbott, against "hero" characters, like Royce and Ken Shamrock, the UFC was becoming more and more like professional wrestling—a stage on which to introduce heroes and heels. It is no coincidence that I only fought professionally in Japan, the home of the samurai and the Bushido code. Like the European knights' concept of chivalry, the Bushido code governed the conduct of Japan's samurai warriors. To them, being a warrior was not just an occupation but a way of life. The tenets of the code changed slightly over time, but they can generally be described as righteousness, courage, compassion, respect, honesty, honor, and loyalty.

My belief in Jiu Jitsu required me to fight in order to validate my teaching to my students. It was important that I expose myself to danger and put it all on the line the same way I forced them to do in my academy. This meant, of course, that there was a great deal of weight on my shoulders. I would do my best to win, but I couldn't worry too much about it or I'd risk changing the way I fought.

Worse than the violence and physical punishment of the actual fight was the lonely hell of training for a professional fight. I never lose sight of the fact that I am the one who jumps over the top rope and into the ring. If I depend too much on the love of the fans or the guidance of a coach, I am not fully integrated with myself and cannot harness all of my power.

During the months of strenuous training before a professional fight, I venture deeper and deeper inside myself as the day of the fight grows closer. Even though I trained regularly at the Pico Academy, much of my prefight preparation consisted of brutal cardio and bodyweight exercises. Some of it was based on what I had learned from Orlando Cani, but much of it was just old-fashioned hard work. I was more afraid of the sand dunes near Point Mugu than any of my training partners. I ran up and down those dunes, over and over, my car as my only witness.

Prior to any fight or even big Jiu Jitsu tournaments in Brazil, I would go into nature before them. This became especially important for me in the coming years in Japan. When Yori Nakamura offered me his family's mountain cabin in Karuizawa, near Nagano, to use as a training camp before the Japan Open, I jumped at the opportunity. With the hard training over, I wanted to go to Japan weeks before the fight, get over the jet lag, train in the thin mountain air, and above all, get in sync with the samurai spirit. There was no better place to do this than Karuizawa.

When I was training in California, I had many training partners and others around to help. Once in Japan, however, the group around me shrank and usually consisted of just Royler, Rockson, and Kim. I was extremely selective about whom I wanted around me. My body was a well-oiled machine by that point, and I couldn't risk getting hurt. My emotional and spiritual preparation was equally important.

Each day Royler, Rockson, and I exercised and ate well

before I went into the woods alone and got mentally prepared to go to war. I would usually take my carving tools,
strip the bark off a branch, and shave it until it was clean
and smooth. I liked to do things that required me to focus
completely. Something as simple as cutting a piece of bam-
boo with a knife allowed me to keep my mind on the blade
and to find a rhythm. When I was finished with the stick, I
would add it to the pile of wood that I would burn on my last
day in camp.

A couple of times a week, I would take a snorkel and sub-
merge my entire body in a frozen river. First came the shock
of the cold, followed by searing pain and anxiety, but I got
to a point where I was ready to surrender and die. If you can
control your breathing, you can get past this point to where
the cold disappears and the pain turns to pleasure. In order
to go into water that cold, I had to control myself mentally
and physically. After I emerged from the water and began
to breathe, I was warm despite the freezing temperature. I
didn't even have goosebumps.

On my last day in the mountains, I lit the big pile of wood
and leaves that I collected during my stay. The flames spread
upward quickly until the entire pile was engulfed. I didn't
feed the fire but instead kept my eyes on it the entire time.
I offered my thanks for the opportunity to be there and to
represent Jiu Jitsu. In the thirty minutes that it took for the
fire to start and then burn itself out, I saw my entire life play
out in front of me. By the time it went out, I had prayed, rid
myself of any doubts or regrets, and accepted the cycle of

life and death. Afterward, I felt ready to kill or be killed, and knew that I could flow from a clinch to a throw to a choke to whatever the situation required, with total confidence. I knew that I could overcome any obstacle and capitalize on the first opportunity.

This ritual was my final and most important divine meditation, part of the process of pulling even further away from my team of supporters and going inside myself. I embraced loneliness because it would give me the strength I needed later on. My rational mind would be turned off until the fights were over.

In the beginning, the Japanese were extremely curious about me, but they were also skeptical because they believed that their pro wrestlers were invincible. When I walked into the press conference in Tokyo, one of the Japanese reporters asked, "Where have you been? Some people worried that you might miss the fight." When I told him that I had been in the mountains near Nagano, he looked confused. Then I told him that I wanted to be in a peaceful place to focus on the fight and connect with the spirit of the samurai, to which he responded with an even more confused look. Another reporter asked me what my strategy was for the fight, and I told him that it was impossible to say, because I would capitalize on my opponent's weaknesses in the moment and seize whatever opportunities he gave me. It was impossible to predict where my mind and body would take me.

Unlike the UFC, the Japan Open had gloves and twenty-minute rounds. Because it was an eight-man tournament,

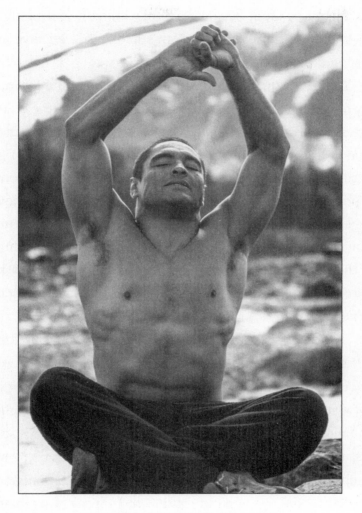

RICKSON GRACIE PREPARES FOR BATTLE.
PHOTOGRAPH COURTESY OF SUSUMU NAGAO.

the winner would have to fight three bouts in one night. I would have to keep an open mind. I couldn't go in with a strategy or plan, because I didn't know who'd be fighting me. My solutions to problems had to be reflexive and responsive.

To me, my fights were solemn celebrations, and I wanted my family, friends, and students there to witness the culmination of all the training, all the sacrifice, and all the hard work. On the morning of the Japan Vale Tudo Open, I got to the stadium early and took a long nap in the locker room. When I woke up, I thanked God for life and then acknowledged that it was a perfect day to die because my life's mission was complete. I was representing my art and my family in the ring. My opponent would have to knock me out or kill me to win, for I was never going to tap. This was not a sport to me; it was my sacred honor.

Before I left my dressing room, I put a shell around myself so that I was protected from all unnecessary external information and the emotions of others. I didn't want tunnel vision, but rather a feeling of emptiness, peace of mind, and resignation to my fate so that nothing could surprise or disturb me. The only thing that mattered at that point was jumping into the ring and being alone with my opponent.

Next, I did my workout routine and got my heart racing. Finally, I meditated and began to breathe with the goal of bringing my heart rate down to 60 beats per minute. As the pace of the fight escalated, my opponent would have to rest before me, and that was when I would go for the kill. My window of opportunity in a fight could be something as small as a badly timed exhalation.

My approach to fighting and life was always smart. Above all, it was about being comfortable and mentally in charge and leading my opponent where I wanted him to go. If you are uncomfortable, you are losing. Depending on how you struggle, I will capitalize. While I like the sniper's motto, "One shot, one kill," my situation is different from the sniper's because I don't have the luxury of distance. What I do is much more intimate than killing someone with a rifle from hundreds of yards away.

I was never sure how I was going to kill, but I was always sure that I could cause the kind of discomfort that causes panic. If I am mounted on you, you are going to feel uncomfortable immediately. If you are mounted on me, I will never let you relax enough to feel comfortable because you will be too busy trying to defend my *upa* (neck-bridge) and my elbow escape. I will make sure that you are unstable and reacting so that my actions will dictate the terms of the fight.

My first fight in the fifty-thousand-person arena was against a Japanese judoka named Yoshinori Nishi. In most fights there comes a time when a window of opportunity opens and you must recognize and seize it. In this fight, mine came before the bell had even rung. After I jumped into the ring, I looked into Nishi's eyes and then at his posture. I saw no fire, no viciousness, no aggression. Nishi looked lost, as though he was trying to remember a play from a playbook.

The bell rang and I walked toward him—not in a fighting stance but as if I was crossing a park. I immediately sensed Nishi's confusion. He didn't know if I was coming to shake his hand, kiss him, or punch him. By the time he realized it, I had bridged the gap, it was too late to hit me, we were in a clinch, and he was headed to the ground with me on top of him. Worse than the fact that he was now on the ground, his playbook had gone out the window, and he was completely lost. A few punches later, my opponent turned his back, I sank a choke, and the fight was over in less than three minutes.

My second fight was against a six-five, 275-pound Wing Tsun fighter named David Levicki. When I saw him in the hallway before the event, I walked over to him and shook his hand out of respect. He jokingly said to me, "If you get my arm, please don't break it." I was stunned and felt I'd won the fight before it started. His cornerman and coach, Gerard Gordeau, the Dutch kickboxer who bit Royce in the first UFC, was as mean as a snake, but Levicki was not.

I got into the ring with David, who looked afraid and didn't want to engage. The American was more focused on surviving than winning. Although he had a huge reach advantage and I am not a striker, I started trying to punch him to close the distance and get him on the ground. I got Levicki in a clinch and started to take him down, but we fell out of the ring. He landed on top of me on the concrete below. The second we hit the hard ground, I reversed the position, got on top, and kept attacking him.

The referees separated us, and I jumped right back into the ring. I could have been severely injured by the fall, and now I wanted to quickly finish this fight. The big American was slow to get up and seemed reluctant to get back into the ring. When he finally climbed back in, I took him to the ground again and mounted, but rather than punching him, I smashed his lower back with my knee. With each blow, I could feel the will to fight leaving him. Even with Gordeau shouting instructions—he was totally lost. Before I could even sink a choke, Levicki tapped out.

I faced a tall American kickboxer named Bud Smith in the finals. The second the bell rang he threw a weak front kick that I caught and used to throw him on his back. Twenty unanswered punches later, Smith also tapped out. In three short bouts, I had won the Japan Open. I bowed to the crowd on the four sides of the ring but did not smile. The samurai did not celebrate victories, and neither would I. Why celebrate a victory? Your next fight might be your last. Battles are not parties. Win or lose, fights are sacred to me.

When the ring announcer thrust the microphone into my face, I made sure to thank him first in Japanese, and then I told the crowd that I was honored to win in Japan, the home of the samurai and the place where Jiu Jitsu originated. The Japanese understood my attitude and code of honor perfectly. Not only had a martial art, taught to my family by one of Japan's greatest fighters, come home, but I had also showed them that the Bushido code had not been lost on the Gracie family.

In less than six minutes of fighting, Jiu Jitsu had defeated kickboxing, Kung Fu, and, most important, wrestling. Winning the first Japan Open was one of the great triumphs of my life. But perhaps even greater was the knowledge that the Japanese crowd and I connected on a profound level that night. Even today, the Japanese people treat me with great respect because I respected and upheld their warrior tradition.

After the Japan Vale Tudo Open, the Japanese fans got interested in MMA and wondered how their wrestling idols would do against a fighter like me. Soon the Japanese wrestling magazines started to speculate about which pro wrestler was going to kick my ass. When I got back to LA, I learned that one of Japan's most famous pro wrestlers, Nobuhiko Takada, had challenged me. Takada was an owner of one of the most popular pro wrestling leagues in Japan (Union of Wrestling Forces International), and I figured that he was trying to use me for a publicity stunt.

I ignored him and took my family to Fiji's Tavarua Island for two weeks of surfing. We had taken a big chance by breaking away from Rorion. We had pulled it off, and now it was time to celebrate. "Cloudbreak," the open-ocean wave near the island, was powerful and could be intimidating when it got big. I suffered some bad wipeouts, but toward the end of our trip, I surfed the best waves of my life. It was a joyful time for all of us, and we returned to LA reenergized and inspired.

A few weeks after we returned, my representative in Japan called to tell me that Takada was telling the press that I had not responded to him because I was afraid to fight.

I wrote a press release about Takada's challenge and stated very clearly that I refused to fight fixed fights and would never step into a professional wrestling ring. However, if Takada wanted to fight in the next Japan Open or even on the street, I looked forward to it.

A week later, Takada's protégé, Yoji Anjo, one of the villains of Japanese pro wrestling, held a press conference in Tokyo to announce that he was traveling to Los Angeles to fight me *to the death*. When I heard that Anjo had said this, I told him to call me when he got to town. I wasn't going to stress out about it. If Anjo came to fight, then we'd fight. The Japanese promoters and reporters were always creating dramas and then fanning the flames. These kinds of theatrics were the story of my life by then; I never lost sleep over barking dogs. I compartmentalized the threats.

On the morning of December 7, 1994, the fifty-third anniversary of the Japanese attack on Pearl Harbor, I received a call from Luis "Limão" Heredia, the head instructor at the Pico Academy. He told me that a dozen Japanese reporters with cameras, a pro wrestling official, and a pro wrestler were at the academy demanding to see me.

I taped my hands as I drove down the Pacific Coast Highway. Whether he realized it or not, Yoji Anjo was now in very deep water. If I'm fighting for money, I'll stop hitting you when you or the referee asks me to. If we are fighting for honor, I'll stop hitting you when I feel like it. Yoji Anjo invaded my academy and disrespected me in front of my students. I needed to make an example out of him.

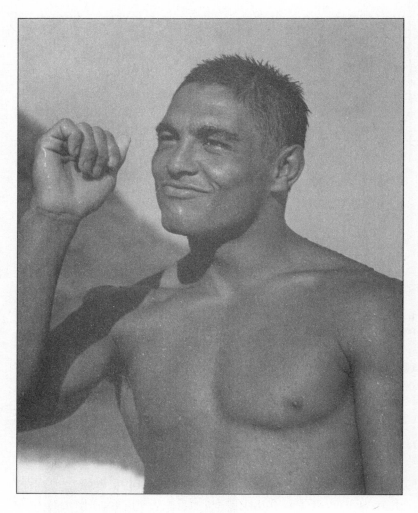

RICKSON GRACIE, RIO.
PHOTOGRAPH COURTESY OF BRUCE WEBER.

I pulled down the driveway of the Pico Academy and saw Japanese reporters with cameras crowded outside the door. I walked inside and saw a Japanese guy in a flashy suit next to a woman in a fancy dress. I greeted them politely and asked them what they wanted. The man in the suit was Shinji Sasazaki, a former wrestler who was now a pro wrestling official. He flashed me a fake smile and said that he had come to invite me to fight in their league in Japan. "Thanks, but I don't fight fixed fights and will never fight in a pro wrestling league," I replied.

Then Sasazaki looked at me seriously and said, "You also said that you would be willing to fight for free for your honor?"

When I asked him if he had come to fight or negotiate he said, "Our fighter is outside. Can he come in?" I told Limão and my students to let the fighter in but to keep all of the reporters out. Yoji Anjo marched into my academy and gave me a dirty look. There was a scuffle at the door, but the reporters were no match for my students, who pushed them out and closed the door behind them.

I am not sure that Anjo was even there to fight. If he could go back to Japan and tell the media, "I went to Rickson Academy to fight, but he wouldn't fight me," that would have been enough. Still, Anjo was confident; I could sense it by the way that he was acting. I handed Anjo an injury waiver to sign, and he scowled and said something to Sasazaki, who asked, "You mean, if he doesn't sign this, you won't fight?" Once again, I felt like I was being set up. If I said "yes," they would go back to Japan and say that I chickened out of the fight. I sensed their malice and said, "No, no forget the paper. If he came to fight, let's fight. The winner gets the videotape."

I took off my T-shirt and stepped onto the mat in the same gray sweatpants I had slept in. Anjo followed me to the center of the mat and we squared off. I threw a leg kick, shot, clinched, and took him to the ground. When I mounted, Anjo stuck his index finger in my mouth, and tried with all of his might to poke it through my cheek. There was no way that I was going to turn my head and risk losing my position so I resigned myself to the fact that his finger was going to rip through my cheek. That was OK. It would never stop me.

After a few punches, I removed the fishhook, and now Yoji Anjo needed to pay. At first I was prepared to beat him and send him on his way, but after he fishhooked me, he had escalated this conflict to a new level, and I wanted to fucking kill him. Before I really began to hit him, I took my time moving the wrestler to the center of the mats so he couldn't escape. Then I methodically rained punches down on his face. Anjo tried to turn, probably hoping that I would choke him, but there was no way that I was going to let him off that easy. I kept punching him until his nose was broken and both of his eyes were swollen shut. Then I choked him unconscious and left him sleeping in the center of my mats in a puddle of his own blood.

I walked to the door that all the reporters were huddled

behind and opened it. As the press streamed into the Pico Academy, Sasazaki lifted Anjo off the mat and tried to cover his bloody face. When the photographers tried to take pictures of him, he knelt in front of Anjo to block their view. Kim walked over to Sasazaki and told him not to cover Anjo's face but to stand up and move away. The Japanese reporters gasped when they saw his bloody, swollen face and his ailing body.

Anjo got off lightly and was lucky that he didn't leave the Pico Academy on a stretcher. After all, when the scientists from National Geographic's television show *Fight Science* measured how much lateral force I could deliver to the atlas, the top vertebra, which connects the skull to the spine, according to their instruments, I generated six hundred foot-pounds of force.

A fight like this was very different from a professional one. My decision to fight or not to fight has never been based on money, prefight hype, or whom I was channeling my anger toward. I am guided by my personal code of honor. Yoji Anjo had come into my school and disrespected me in front of my students, and his punishment needed to be visible for all to see so that nobody could dispute the outcome of this fight. I knew the Japanese would understand this. Imagine if I had shown up unannounced to the Kōdōkan during a class, walked across their sacred tatami mats in my street shoes, and called out the Judo masters!

A few days later, Yoji Anjo returned to the Pico Academy with flowers, a Samurai helmet, and a letter of apology. I thought this was decent of him and figured that he realized the error of his ways and that it was over. A week or so later, however, my manager in Japan called to tell me that when Anjo got home, he told everyone that my students jumped him and beat him up. First, I issued this press release:

On 07 December a UWF [United Wrestling Federation] representative dressed in a black suit and accompanied by his colleague . . . showed up at my studio at approximately eleven o'clock in the morning. They demanded to speak with me. My assistant fearing for the welfare of the students because of the belligerent and antagonistic attitude of the UWF representatives called and told me to come to the studio immediately. When I arrived at the studio, I questioned . . . the representatives as to the reason for their visit. . . . At this point, the UWF representatives then advised me that they did not come to talk about business; they came to fight. I accepted the challenge . . . thinking that the big representative was Takada. . . . I don't have to describe the fight itself because Mr. Anjo's face tells the story of what happened better than words ever could. . . . I don't want to validate the dishonorable acts of the UWF or the foolish acts of Mr. Anjo, but I must say, in this instance, Mr. Anjo did fight for real and he lost like a man. Even though the UWF came to my studio by surprise, I proved to them that I am always ready to fight for my honor. At the current time, I have several fight deals in the plans for the near future. To me, these legitimate endeavors are much more important than any more surprises created by the UWF.

Thank you,
Rickson Gracie

Then I told my representative to set up a press conference in Tokyo where we could show the video of the fight. After the Japanese press watched the video, the fans learned that this was a fair fight and that Anjo had lied. As a result, my reputation grew even larger in Japan. Although the fans still loved me, Japanese pro wrestling did not after I beat Anjo and called them out for fixing fights. Now, there was only one man who could redeem pro wrestling's reputation: Anjo's mentor, Takada, the king of Japanese pro wrestling.

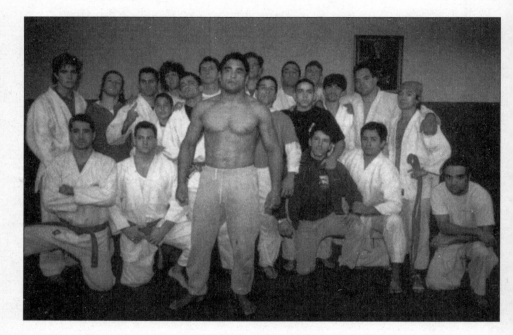

THE PICO ACADEMY AFTER THE ANJO FIGHT.
PHOTOGRAPH COURTESY OF THE RICKSON GRACIE COLLECTION.

PARADIGM SHIFTS

I WAS GETTING READY FOR THE JAPAN OPEN 2 IN EARLY 1995 when I received a call from my dad. He wanted me to meet with him and Rorion to discuss me fighting in the UFC. My star was rising in Japan, but Royce's was falling in the UFC. Even though he came back to win UFC 4, the American fighters were getting wise to his game, especially the wrestlers. Matches that took him two minutes to win a year earlier were now taking him fifteen minutes of hard fighting.

Royce had promised me some of his prize money if I would train and coach him for the UFC. After Royce won, Rorion kept his prize money, and I got nothing. When it came time for Royce to get ready for the second UFC, he made me the same promise. I helped him yet again, and after he won, Rorion kept his winnings and gave me nothing. I was there to support the cause of Jiu Jitsu while Rorion was there to support the cause of, well, Rorion. By the time Rorion, my dad, and UFC president Art Davie finally approached me about fighting in the UFC, my dealings with them were strictly business.

I didn't like the direction the UFC was going. To appease their fans and the American politicians who were now trying to outlaw MMA fighting, the UFC was moving further and further away from the long *vale tudo* matches that I preferred. Royce's days were numbered, and my dad and Rorion knew it.

In the beginning, the UFC was promoting real *vale tudo* fights. Once American politicians began to criticize it, the UFC modified their rules to shorten the rounds and create weight divisions, turning a martial arts contest into a sport. Having only five minutes in a round to capitalize on an opportunity fundamentally changes the nature of a fight. Although the rules make the UFC more entertaining for fans, ironically, they also make it more violent and less strategic and technical. The UFC was transforming *vale tudo* into something more brutal.

When Kim and I met with my dad, Rorion, and Art Davie at an office in Los Angeles, I told them that I would be happy to fight for a million dollars. When Art tried to justify the UFC's paltry pay scale, I told him that this was his problem, not mine. Finally, my dad played the Gracie card and told me that in his day, he fought for family honor, not money. I had done plenty of heavy lifting for my family up until now, but I had my own children to feed. Rorion had no hold over me anymore, and it seemed that many Gracies were rebelling against his rule. America was quickly reshaping our family hierarchy and dynamics. Now it was every Gracie for himself.

By 1995, I was still teaching at the Pico Academy but mostly focused on fighting and defending my title in Japan. If you are the champion and you rely only on your ability, you won't be champion for long. When a champ has only physical ability, he is incomplete. That's the difference between a champion who's stagnating and one who's dynamic. After tennis great Roger Federer lost a few matches and felt that his competition was catching up to him, he reinvented himself. He studied his swing and began to hit the ball closer to the ground. The reason race car driver Ayrton Senna was such an inspiration was that he was a champion whose mind never stopped spinning; he was never content with his performance, even when he was winning.

I've been extremely competitive all my life. If we go to the pool and I lose a race, I'll be back at the pool the next day, and the day after that, to practice. That defeat will stay in my mind until I get a chance to avenge it. The last time I lost in competition, I was a fourteen-year-old orange belt in a small tournament that my dad took some of the younger kids to. I remember it like yesterday. When my match started and we hit the ground, my opponent surprised me with his athleti-cism. Before I realized what was happening, he was on my back and choking me. I tapped out and was so mad at myself that I began to train harder than ever before.

That poor kid who beat me now had a bull's-eye on his head! We faced each other a few months later at another tournament. I beat him, but only by decision, which made me angrier and motivated me to train even harder for our next rematch. Four or five months later, we met again as green belts. When the match started, he put his foot on my hip and caught me in a very smooth armlock. His leg went over my face, my arm stretched, and my elbow hyperextended. Even though I felt my ligaments and tendons popping, I didn't tap. Instead, I freed my arm, got on top, and started to choke him. I kept saying, "Don't tap, motherfucker! Don't tap!" He tapped and never posed a challenge to me again.

After I learned to empty my mind, I had the confidence to be humble, and humility played a big role in my progress. Just because I won the first Japan Open, I didn't rest on my laurels. Instead, I focused on my weaknesses, which allowed me to examine and appreciate minute details that I would have overlooked if I'd had no humility. In order to push my-self, I needed to feel stress, disappointment, and frustration on a daily basis.

I always tried to work from a place of discomfort and would often line up all my students and tell them that I was going to have a match with each of them. If anyone could survive three minutes, they were the winner. The only submission I was allowed was an armlock on their left arm. If I beat nineteen of them, but one guy lasted longer than three minutes, I'd go home feeling sick. That gave me the taste of defeat, and I kept that taste in my mouth at all times by constantly creating challenges that kept me connected with defeat.

Some people train and train but never get any better because they practice only what they're good at against people they can beat. Because they never address their weaknesses, they stop growing, and the competition catches them. Those champions who say, "Fuck, I'm just going to keep doing what I do well," eventually falter because natural talent can take you only so far. If you don't understand yourself, how effective can you be at anything?

You also cannot become a great warrior by memorizing Sun Tzu or Miyamoto Musashi, because fighting is both an art *and* a science. It is artistic because it requires creativity, passion, and instinct. It is scientific because there are empirical aspects like technique, timing, strength, and endurance that also cannot be ignored. Sometimes my cornerman might tell me to move right, but I might say to myself, "Fuck right, I'm going left." I'm the one in the ring. I can see and sense things that no one else can and so must trust my instincts.

I never thought in the ring; I felt. At the peak of my career, my senses were so finely tuned that I could smell my opponent's fear and watch him leak energy. Because of this sensitivity, I never fought blind or tried to force opportunities. Instead, I established a connection with my opponent and either waited for a mistake or solved whatever problem he presented. In either case, I was able to act or react with total commitment because my mind had been emptied of expectations so my reactions were spontaneous.

The champion wrestlers, judokas, and kickboxers who succeeded in MMA, people like Ronda Rousey, Randy Couture, and Bas Rutten, were all established champions who knew how to train and fight long before they stepped into the cage. It's no coincidence that Ronda Rousey was once the most dominant fighter in the world. She was a unique fighter who could manage stress and had an amazing work ethic; the whole formula was there. Her domination in MMA was not due to size, strength, or luck but was the result of perfect technique that she executed brutally.

For a time, Ronda's movements came from her deep subconscious, and she fought on autopilot. She reached a point that is beyond knowledge because she was a martial artist, as opposed to a jack-of-all-trades, master-of-none MMA fighter. Not only was she an Olympic medalist; she was a judo master and the daughter of a judo master. Ronda Rousey was on a different level than her competition. She was playing chess, while they were playing checkers. Then she got distracted by show business, drifted away from grappling, trained however she felt like training, and lost her way.

I sensed trouble when Ronda's focus shifted from fighting to becoming a public personality and capitalizing on it. The life of an elite athlete and the life of a celebrity are very different. I met Ronda while she was the UFC champ and was on top of the world. My only advice to her was to focus on fighting and have someone insulate and protect her from the media circus. If you pay too much attention to the media and the things other people expect from you, not only will you lose focus, but you will also lose the sensitivity you need in the cage. Every fight requires your full attention because your opponents are not distracted. They are in the gym every day trying to figure out how to beat you.

Ronda Rousey was not exactly receptive to my advice and acted as though nobody had anything to teach her. In the end, she got so lost and so far off track that she tried to stand toe to toe with a world champion boxer. After Holly Holm knocked her out, she needed a sensible and honest explanation as to why she lost so badly, as well as a new plan of attack in order to put this behind her and move forward. Shattering disappointments require you to be radically honest with yourself, a process that can be painful but is absolutely necessary. If people provide you with excuses and encourage you to double down on your failed strategy, you will have ghosts living inside your head that will come out to haunt you at the worst possible times.

Because so much of Ronda's identity was tied to being the UFC champion, losing was especially hard for her. After she got knocked out, nobody addressed her most obvious and fundamental strategic problem—she's not a striker! If I were fighting Maurice Smith, I would never stand in the middle of the ring and trade blows with him. I would carefully take him to the ground and make him fight my fight.

In the end, Ronda doubled down on her failed strategy. She tried to stand toe to toe with Amanda Nunes, another scary world champion boxer, and got knocked out in less than a minute! Ronda Rousey did not just lose; she was defeated. She never fought MMA again but retreated to the safer, shallower waters of professional wrestling.

My brother Royce did a similar thing when he fought Wallid Ismail in Brazil in a Jiu Jitsu match. Even though Royce was the UFC champ, he had been away from competitive Jiu Jitsu for years and did not take the match very seriously. Wallid, on the other hand, woke up when it was still dark, ran on the beach, and trained in the heat of the day against the toughest guys in Brazil. Sure, Wallid had a limited arsenal, but he had a huge heart. I remember when he fought one of my students in a tournament and my student caught him in a triangle. Wallid spent five minutes in it, and even though his face turned purple and blood was pouring from his nose, he refused to tap! Eventually he escaped and won the fight. When Royce fought Wallid, he thought that he was going to give a demonstration, but he got choked unconscious instead.

Some fighters are not overconfident but try to fight from a place of anger. Whenever there was a big Jiu Jitsu tournament in LA, I would go and personally invite the top black belts to come and train at my academy. A top Jiu Jitsu competitor and MMA fighter took me up on my invitation. I was curious about him because sometimes he fought great, but other times he just fell apart. When I first shook his hand and looked into his eyes, I could see and feel how emotionally uncentered he was. After I beat him fairly easily, he stuck around for a few days to train with me. What I noticed most about him was that although his Jiu Jitsu was technically excellent, he could not apply it to his life off the mat. This fighter took drugs instead of finding a more holistic way to balance himself, which only made him more uncentered. He was a superficial warrior who lacked the spiritual component. Years later, I saw the same fighter coaching a young MMA fighter in a bout in Japan. When the fight began and his fighter started to feel out his opponent, he began to scream at him, "Get in there and start trading punches! Don't be a fucking pussy!" He was trying to goad his fighter on an emotional level by publicly humiliating him and making him feel like a coward. The young fighter attacked blindly, exhausted himself, and lost the fight. No surprise there.

The mental part of the game is the most challenging. Even Rockson, my own son, could never grasp aspects of it. Rockson used to say that his goal was to be as good as or better than me. Although these were basically the same goals I had at his age, the way we pursued them could not have been more different. He was so intent on filling my shoes that he pushed himself too hard. Rockson always wanted to accelerate things; nothing ever happened fast enough for him. His gas pedal was always floored. He would never stop and wait for his opponent to make a mistake—just offense, offense, offense. When Rockson competed in tournaments, he would attack his opponent like a tornado. Defense, patience, counters—no way. He would escalate the fight quickly and go for submissions even when they were not there. I would say, "Calmo! Calmo!" over and over, but it did no good.

Rockson had all of the tools and resources at his fingertips to be the best. In addition to my knowledge, the best training partners, and the support of his family, he also had the passion and drive. If he had used his Jiu Jitsu in a more conceptual way—by employing timing, connection, weight distribution, pressure—he would have gotten much better results. Yes, Rockson was fearless and courageous, but unlike me, he never calculated risks and kept getting even more reckless. Worse, he continued to drift toward the dark side.

Sometimes Rockson would come home with new DVD players or the latest video games. When I asked where he got them, he would say, "I found it on the street." One day a policeman who knew me called and said, "I have Rockson here. We caught him trying to steal from a store. You need to come down." When I arrived, my son was sitting on the curb. "Rickson, I'm not going to take him in," the cop said, "but talk to him. He could have gotten into serious trouble." When I lectured Rockson on the drive home about how it was wrong to steal and that he didn't need to do so in order to prove his worth, he remained silent and stared at his feet. When we got home, I said, "Go to the garage, I'm not finished talking to you." He looked me dead in the eyes and groaned, "Dad, can't you just hit me? I'd rather you do that than more talking. We don't need to talk anymore—just give me my punishment." I thought, *Fuck, what am I going to do to make him fear the consequences of his actions?* That was when I realized that I was losing control of my son. Rockson reminded me of my brother Rolls, in that they both possessed psychologies that made me uncomfortable. But while this worried me, I figured that it was a phase that he would pass through, as I had. At that time, most of my focus was on defending my title at the second Japan Open.

When I returned to Japan in 1995, a few weeks before the tournament, I went to Yori Nakamura's mountain cabin in Karuizawa. My prefight routine was the same. The hard work was over, and my biggest concern was getting acclimated to Japan without getting hurt or sick. By now, Nagano prefecture felt like my spiritual home. The more time I spent in Japan, the more I liked it. I was amazed by the attention the Japanese paid to the tiniest details of the simplest things: the way they built a fence, the way they planted a garden, the way they turned buckwheat into soba noodles. There is beauty even in their approach to war. Not only do they uphold the values of honor, dignity, and respect, but their weapons, armor, and masks are all beautifully and meticulously constructed. Samurai swords from hundreds of years ago are still some of the finest knives ever made.

Once I got to the mountains, I fell into an easy routine, and by the time I left, I felt that I had cleared and sharpened my mind. My opponents in the second Japan Open were a cross-section of wrestlers and strikers and included Gerard Gordeau, the Dutch kickboxer who bit Royce's ear in a UFC match. I knew the Dutchman was vicious and not interested in a fair or honorable bout. If the referee wasn't looking, he would go for the eyes, or bite. If I fought him, it was going to be with total viciousness, but I did not waste time or energy thinking about it.

My first fight was against a Japanese wrestler named Yoshihisa Yamamoto. When the fight began, we engaged and went into a corner. Yamamoto grabbed the ropes. He was strong and willing to eat punch after punch to avoid going to the ground. I delivered unanswered punches for almost six minutes, but toward the end of the round, Yamamoto grabbed my head, put me in a guillotine choke, used the rope for leverage, and cranked my neck. I tensed up and felt a burst of pain in my neck. After I got my head and neck free, I pushed and kicked Yamamoto out of the ring.

This wrestler was the first fighter to survive a round with me, and he enthused the Japanese crowd. In the second round, he continued to hang on to the ropes, take my shots, and try to catch me in guillotines and kimuras. In the third round—longer than I had fought in a long time—I stayed in the center of the ring and forced Yamamoto to come to me. Like most wrestlers, he was an unskilled striker, so I hit him with a few stiff jabs. When he tried to retreat to the corner and grab the ropes, I disengaged and returned to the center of the ring. I kept punching him in the face, and when his nose began to bleed, I started kicking him in the knees and legs. I noticed that Yamamoto kept touching his nose. I sensed that he was tired and overwhelmed. This was my window of opportunity. I took him down, mounted, and when he turned his back, I choked him unconscious.

I got back to the locker room and could feel that something was wrong with my neck. I did not have 100 percent of my strength and would have to fight around the injury in my next bout against another big Japanese wrestler, named Koichiro Kimura. When the fight began, Kimura shot for a single-leg takedown, and because of my injured neck, I couldn't sprawl properly to avoid it. I let him lift me high into the air and think that he was going to slam me. But because I was totally connected to him and his movement, I used Kimura's energy to spin in the air, and I landed on my feet facing my opponent. From there I took his back and submitted him with a choke. After our fight, Kimura said that he was grateful for the opportunity to fight me and that he was impressed by the depth of Gracie Jiu Jitsu and planned to study it.

I was now in the finals and would face a 155-pound Japanese wrestler named Yūki Nakai, who I was amazed was still fighting. In Nakai's first fight of the night, Gerard Gordeau gouged his eye so badly that he permanently blinded it. Even then, the tiny wrestler persevered, caught Gordeau in an ankle lock, and won. Next Nakai fought a giant American wrestler who outweighed him by a hundred pounds and threw him around the ring for twenty minutes before Nakai caught him in an armlock. He, too, tapped out.

After he beat the American, he began screaming, "Rickson, I'm coming for you!"

Yūki was a brave man, and his display of heart was something I will never forget. When I told my team in the locker room before the fight that I wasn't going to hit this badly wounded warrior, there was a brief debate between Royler, Sergio, and me.

Rockson: "Did you see that guy's face! The poor guy! Both of his eyes were closed!"

Royler: "You've got to hit him."

Me: "Not even a punch. I won't do it."

Sergio: "This guy is the worst enemy you've ever had in your life! Punch him in the face! You punch me, so why not him? Don't feel sorry for this guy."

Even though Sergio and my brother objected to my decision, I could see the relief on my son's face. Rockson had seen Nakai's closed, bloody eye, an eye that he would never see out of again, up close and had nothing but respect and pity for this lionhearted man. I was powerful enough to do whatever I wanted, but I had compassion toward Yūki Nakai.

I tried to make our fight a technical confrontation, nothing too physical or brutal. Based on his display of courage, he was entitled to this. I felt that a technical win against such a badly injured opponent was a much more honorable path to victory. There was no reason to use my power in a capricious way. So what did I do? I beat Yūki Nakai in a five-minute grappling match. Although I won in the ring, I did not break him. His spirit was too strong. Yūki Nakai was the modern samurai that night. True strength, like Yūki's, is not always demonstrated through victory.

With every win, I doubled my price. After I won in 1995, the Japanese told me that they could not meet my demand of $400,000 to show and $400,000 to win. I refused to fight for less money and suggested that my brother Royler do so instead. This would give the Japanese time to come up with the money they needed for me to fight. Of course, I was always ready to fight for my honor, but professional fights were a different matter. Once I signed the contract and the date for the fight was set, there were huge expectations on me. The promoter expected me to fill the Tokyo Dome. My friends, family, and students expected me to win, and the Japanese expected a Japanese fighter to beat me.

I cornered for Royler when he fought Noboru Asahi in Tokyo. When he defeated his Japanese opponent, I jumped into the ring and helped Asahi to his feet. During the post-fight press conference, Royler thanked me for coaching him and arranging this fight for him. Now the Japanese promoters got serious about my next fight. I was 6–0 in Japan and had won every fight by submission.

I was no longer interested in fighting tournaments that required me to beat three opponents in a single night. Moving forward, I would fight only title fights. Some criticize me for fighting "weak" opponents and not taking on the top American fighters of that time. But if anyone wanted to fight me badly enough, all he had to do was show up at my academy. Just ask Yoji Anjo.

By 1996, the Japanese promoters who had spent a great deal of time and money building me up now wanted to take me down. However, it was not as simple as unleashing a smashing machine on me. If the Japanese were going to pay me more than anyone had ever been paid to fight an MMA match, my opponent would have to be Japanese.

Don't get me wrong, the first-generation American wrestlers in MMA impressed me very much. They combined pure strength with great technique and had incredible power. Even though I never fought any of the smashing machines, my mind began to spin after I watched a videotape of a fight between Mark Kerr and my friend and Brazilian Jiu Jitsu champion Fábio Gurgel.

At six three and 260 pounds, with only 5 percent body fat and huge muscles pulsing with steroid strength, Kerr was a physical specimen. Fábio showed great heart in their thirty-minute bout, but the American stayed on top and pounded him with punches and head butts. The morning after I watched the fight, I woke up thinking, *How the fuck would I deal with that monster?* My son Rockson was eighty pounds lighter than me, close to the difference between Kerr and Fábio, so I told him to meet me in the garage.

I had Rockson lie down, and I got inside his guard so that we would start in the position that Mark Kerr beat up Fábio so badly from. At first, I made him uncomfortable, and then helped him adjust: "Rockson, move your hip a little bit, stretch. Move your hip more like this, push like this, use your foot." This was not hard training. I was simply dissecting positions and helping Rockson find ways to deal with my power and alleviate the discomfort of my being on top of him.

I realized that Fábio Gurgel's biggest mistake was that he stayed flat on his back and created no angles. I showed Rockson how to take away my comfort by keeping me off balance. After about forty minutes on the mat, I was confident that I had the tools needed for the job. If I had to fight Kerr tomorrow, I had a chance that I did not have the day before.

My next bout would not be against Kerr. The Japanese promoters wanted me to take on one of their most popular pro wrestlers, Nobuhiko Takada. Our bout would be the main event in the first Pride Fighting Championship. This new promotion was the best MMA league in the world until the UFC bought it. I worked with the Pride officials on the rules so that, unlike the UFC's rules, they were built around the fighters instead of the fans. I wanted to make sure that the referee did not have the power to arbitrarily force fighters on the ground to stand up.

Once the contract was signed and the date was set for October 11, 1997, I began to train in earnest. Often I would ride my bike on the beach path from Pacific Palisades to Santa Monica to warm up. One day, on the way home, I stopped at Will Rogers State Beach to jump into the ocean and cool off. I walked my bike to the edge of the sea, and as I was taking off my shoes, I noticed something white poking through the sand. I didn't know if it was a rock or a shell, but I immediately felt drawn to it, so I dug it out.

It was a small wooden figure with the head of an elephant

and human arms and legs. It looked vaguely familiar, and for whatever reason, I felt its positive energy in the same way that I felt drawn to the energy of the sun or the sea. I put it into my pocket and took it home. When I got home, I felt compelled to build the figurine a small house in my backyard. First, I made a wooden floor, then I built a frame that I thatched with palm fronds. Once I was satisfied with how it looked, I put the statue inside. I do not believe in luck or coincidence; to me, everything is a sign that is either positive or negative. I accept the fact that forces larger than me are in charge, and I look for spiritual clues in life. For example, if I find a hawk feather in my garden, I consider it a blessing and a good sign.

My spirituality is based on things that I cannot explain but nonetheless believe. Americans tend to be hyperrational: everything must fit into the right box, and all of the dots must connect. When I moved to the US, it was much harder for me to express myself spiritually and to capture the energy that transcends the rational. People here live according to what they can prove and explain. If they can't explain something, they deem it unacceptable and unbelievable. However, rationality has its limits; not everything can be explained on paper. Just look into the sky on a clear night. Where does the universe begin? Where does it end? Are we the only form of life in it? Is there life after death? Simple questions without easy answers.

Even though most Brazilians are Catholic, they still believe in mystical powers and notions that cannot be explained scientifically or rationally. Macumba, voodoo, black magic, spiritual mediums—although their ceremonies and practices differ, most of these traditions involve an attempt to contact spirits and get them to help, and sometimes harm, others. Growing up, I would sometimes see the headless chickens that had been used in the previous night's ceremony, and shrines with candles, flowers, and liquor. A close friend's mother was a medium who would receive messages from dead people.

When Kim's brother, Roberto, was in the final stages of cancer, he was undergoing chemotherapy and going downhill fast. He had little left to lose, so he went to a spiritual surgeon in São Paolo. Some of them use a Shiatsu style of massage, others channel energy like Qigong, and some even claim to perform surgeries with kitchen knives. When Roberto went back to the hospital for his next chemo session, the doctor was stunned by his test results and said, "Your numbers look really good. I don't understand how, but they've stabilized. Let's wait on the next chemo session until we see next week's test numbers." Roberto's test results kept getting better and better. The doctor thought that something was wrong with the test, but when he double-checked, he saw that the figures were accurate. After Roberto visited the spiritual doctor, he never had another chemotherapy session; he is still alive today.

Above all, I believe in energy. When I learned that the statuette I had found was of Ganesh, Hindu elephant-god of good fortune, the remover of obstacles, I added an altar to his house. I felt virtuous, having respected what I found before I even knew what it was. A few days later, I left for Japan to fight Takada.

Pride Fighting Championship was not just a sports event promoted by a television network; it was at least partially sponsored by the yakuza. The word *yakuza* actually refers to a worthless hand (ya = 8, ku = 9, za = 3) in a Japanese card game called *oicho-kabu*. Over time, the definition has changed to mean "gambling people," and then organized crime.

While sports events generate revenue from ticket sales and television contracts, the real money is in gambling. In addition to prostitution, extortion, and smuggling, the yakuza was involved in many different types of gambling. With gambling still illegal in Japan, members of different yakuza syndicates served as bookmakers, and one of their favorite sports to gamble on was Sumo wrestling. Different yakuza groups owned Sumo gyms, sponsored fighters, and promoted matches. MMA now offered unique new gambling opportunities, and Hiromichi Momose, a yakuza boss who had spent years in prison, was quick to realize this.

Momose was rumored to have put up ¥50 million for the first Pride event and was a big supporter of Takada. Even though I didn't underestimate Takada, I knew the difference between pro wrestling, a choreographed performance in which you and your opponent work together to put on a good show, and *vale tudo*. I knew that he would find things much more difficult when there was no script to follow.

After my fight camp in the mountains, I felt ready when

I arrived in Tokyo. I stepped into the ring with Takada and did not sense aggression when our fight began. He seemed reluctant to engage. I chased him around the ring for over a minute and then decided to go to the center and make him come to me. We traded some kicks, clinched, and just as I was taking him down, Takada grabbed the rope so the referee would separate and restart us. This irritated me, but I didn't want to get sidetracked by anger, because I saw that Takada was just trying to survive. He was out of his depth, and it was only a matter of time before he made a fatal error.

I turned up the heat, secured a double leg takedown, and slammed Takada on his back. I mounted him and began to punch him in the body and the head. When he tried to grab me with his arm, I arm-barred him. The fight was over in less than five minutes but was a great success: in addition to the more than forty-seven thousand fans who packed the Tokyo Dome, many more watched it on pay-per-view television.

After the Takada fight, a yakuza boss who owned a Sumo wrestling stable invited me to have dinner with him. He was curious about me. I think he wondered how a Brazilian could embody what many in the twentieth century considered outdated Japanese values. I was curious too, and had been amazed by the power the yakuza had in Japan. They would stop and park in the middle of a busy street, and the police didn't dare say a word. A Mercedes sedan pulled up to the Four Seasons, a big driver got out, opened the back door for Kim and me, and then opened the front passenger door for my son Rockson. Just as we started to drive away from the

197

hotel, Rockson noticed that our driver was missing parts of two fingers and asked him how he had lost them. The driver looked at Rockson gravely and said, "I made a mistake."

At dinner, when Kim complimented the yakuza boss on his beautiful diamond earring, he turned to me and said, "Mr. Gracie, if you don't mind, I'd like to give it to your wife." I thanked him, said that it was fine, and he handed Kim the diamond. Before we left, the yakuza boss presented me with a 350-year-old samurai sword. What I remember most vividly from that night was the tempura that the yakuza boss's private chef cooked us. It was one of the most delicious things that I have ever eaten in my life.

I respected the Japanese relationship with food. It was not just the food; it was also the reverence they showed for their seasonal ingredients. The Japanese term *washoku*, which means "Japanese harmony of food," is based around Japan's four seasons and their harvests. For example, you might eat green peas and clams in the spring, shishito peppers and certain types of fish in the summer, mushrooms and eels in the fall, and greens and other types of fish in the winter. Even rice has a season: rice harvested in the early fall is considered the best. There are special plates and bowls for each season. The diner's senses and the overall experience are as important as the food. Every aspect of the meal is a celebration of both sustenance and the season. This attention to detail really humbled me.

I was especially impressed by the Buddhist temples and Shinto shrines. What amazed me most about the temples was how they were constructed with complex joints instead of nails. Not only did the master carpenters who built them match the wood grains; they treated wood like something that was still alive. My guide in Kyoto was a Buddhist monk, so he was able to take me to places that were off-limits for most visitors and even arranged for us to have tea with one of the head monks. After we finished tea, the senior monk took off his prayer beads and gave them to me. I had nothing to give him, so I took off my shirt and handed it to him as a sign of respect.

I returned to California just as my old teacher Orlando Cani happened to be passing through LA on his way to India. I invited him into my house and took him to the backyard to show him Ganesh and the house that I had built for him. I told him that I fished him out of the sand at the beach near my house, and he said, "This is unbelievable and not an accident." I noticed that Ganesh's house was starting to fall apart, so I decided to build him a new one inspired by the temples of Kyoto. I bought some beautiful red pine, got out my carving tools, and began to work with great focus and a newfound sense of purpose. After I finished, I planted white geraniums around Ganesh's new house. I told my physical therapist about the new house I had built, and she told me that if a person wanted to ask something of Ganesh, they needed to first present him with a gift. Without realizing it, I had already given him a present.

I was not expecting to fight Takada again, but the promoter wanted to give him the opportunity for revenge, and so did his fans. I had received $600,000 for the first fight and would get $1.2 million for the second. The money was much more than anyone else was making at the time, and I agreed. By 1997, my overhead was very high. My family's lifestyle had changed dramatically in a few short years. Fighting in Japan enabled us to move from Torrance to the more affluent beachside suburb of Pacific Palisades, where we bought a beautiful house with a pool, a view of the ocean, and easy access to surf. I also opened a new, state-of-the-art academy in Pacific Palisades. My kids were in private schools and I was finally able to buy new cars for Kim and me. All this cost a great deal of money. I was learning that life in America was much more expensive and complicated than life in Brazil. Cars needed to be registered and insured, and tickets needed to be paid on time. If my kids misbehaved in school, the principal called us in to meet with him. As my kids grew up, it got harder to just focus on my training and fighting.

Three and a half months before my second fight with Takada, I hurt my back. I considered canceling the fight but instead went to Brazil to see a physical therapist I knew and trusted. For a month I stretched, iced, worked out in a pool, got deep-tissue massages, and undertook every other form of physical therapy you could imagine. By the time I left Rio, I felt much better, and even though my body was not 100 percent, I decided to fight.

When we got to Japan, my brother Royler, my friend Renato Barretto, Rockson, Kim, and I went to the mountains. On the first day, I began to train for the first time in more than four months. Within minutes, I felt a twinge of pain in my back and stopped immediately. I told Royler that we would only grapple on the ground with no big movements that would have the potential to make my injury worse. Rather than try to push through the pain, I thought it was better for me to feel no pain until the day of the fight. In the mountains we ran, rode bikes, and did some very light work on the mats, but I insisted on no stand-up grappling, throwing, and clinching.

One day when we were walking on the mountain, I saw a golden eagle fly by and then soar above us. When I first noticed it, I pointed it out to the guys and said, "This is a great sign! Eagles are amazing hunters and have incredible eyesight and senses." Soon visits from the golden eagle were part of our routine. Every other day we would be running in the mountains and the same eagle would soar above us with its regal six-foot wingspan. When the eagle made a high-pitched cry, we all got very excited. By the end of our stay, I had formed a strong connection with that bird.

The day I was leaving for the fight in Tokyo, everyone departed before me. I was alone on the second floor of our house in the mountains when I looked out the window and saw the golden eagle sitting on a branch of a big pine tree twenty yards from me. I froze and we locked eyes. For the minute or so that we stared at each other, I felt I was drawing energy from this majestic creature, that the eagle had come to give me one last show of support before the fight. I went to get the camera to get a picture but by the time I got back, the bird was gone. I realized that this special gift was meant for me and for me alone, and I felt energized by this.

Even though I had not trained hard for months, I felt good on the day of the fight. I was told later that Yoji Anjo was in Takada's corner playing his villain wrestling character, but I was so focused on Takada that I didn't notice him. I was trying to detect any weakness or stress but instead sensed a more confident fighter. He reminded me of Hugo Duarte before our second fight. Takada had a plan that he believed would help him solve the Rickson Gracie puzzle. He was ready to fight with all of his heart.

When the bell rang, Takada threw a flurry of punches. None of them landed squarely, but he did manage to fend off my opening attack. It was now clear to me that Takada would not make the same mistakes he had made in the first fight. We grappled on our feet for much of the fight, and with his background as a wrestler, Takada did this well, but I knew that he was using a great deal of energy. After about six minutes, I noticed that his chest was heaving and he was breathing hard. When he tried to rest, I picked up the pace.

Takada was much better prepared, had a better game plan, and had improved his striking and stand-up, but he was still out of his depth. Professional wrestling does not stress fighters the same way that an MMA match does because the two wrestlers work together to choreograph a spectacle with prearranged results. They give each other time to rest and are not accustomed to the continuous struggle of a real bout.

About six minutes into the fight, I was able to drag

Takada down to the mat and into my guard. Again he tried to rest, but I did not let him. I threw punches to his head and heel kicks to his body. Up to this point, Takada had fought a smart match, but he made a fatal error when he grabbed my ankle and attempted a basic ankle lock. I escaped, then reversed the position and was now on top. Once I started going from mount to side control and back to mount, I sensed that Takada was drowning.

I turned up the heat even more, and after a few more punches, he left his arm exposed. I caught him in an armlock, and he tapped out. After the fight, the ring announcer thrust a microphone in my face, and I told the crowd that the founder of Gracie Jiu Jitsu was a Japanese fighter named Mr. Conde Koma (Hideyo Maeda) who taught my family in the beginning of the century. "So I am bringing back the spirit of the samurai my family took from the real samurai Mr. Koma. I am very pleased to stay here and spend great time here in Japan, especially with the food."

Takada was respectful afterward. He thanked me for giving him a rematch and complimented me on my warrior spirit. He had plenty of courage, but he lacked the knowledge to make a seamless transition into the new universe of MMA. My opponent had spent too many years as a professional wrestler, and it had conditioned him for a different kind of conflict.

Throughout the fight and even afterward, my back felt absolutely fine. When I got back to LA, I went to visit Ganesh to thank him. I had been gone for a month, and the first thing that I noticed was that all of the geraniums I had planted had turned from white to red. Ganesh really felt like a friend and ally now, and I took this as a sign that it was time to get back into top fighting shape.

I had dodged a bullet with my back injury, and it was dawning on me that I couldn't fight forever. By 1999, my back, my hip, and other parts of my body were starting to wear out after four decades of fighting, and I had to preserve what I had left because I knew that my next fight would be a big one. The Japanese are fierce competitors and hate to lose. After Takada's much better showing in the second fight, they thought that it was only a matter of time before they could find a Japanese fighter who could beat me.

In just five years, *vale tudo* had morphed into MMA. Even though Gracie Jiu Jitsu had forced a paradigm shift in martial arts, now *everyone* was studying Jiu Jitsu. Many MMA fighters were studying Jiu Jitsu just to learn how to fight against it. To me, *vale tudo* is different from MMA because there are many more possibilities, both good and bad. Until an opportunity presents itself, one has to fight defensively, as Royce did against Dan Severn in UFC 4. Severn weighed 260 pounds and was on top of my brother for sixteen minutes before Royce caught him in a triangle choke from his back. According to today's rules, Royce could never have won that fight. The ref would have stood them up again after five minutes on the ground.

MMA is a game; *vale tudo* is a war. If the rounds are five minutes, you can go 100 percent, because you know that in five minutes you're going to get a few minutes to recover. You build an entire strategy around that break. You also know that your opponent is in your weight division, so he can't radically overpower you as he could if he were fifty pounds heavier than you.

The environment I'm most comfortable in is one without weight divisions, time limits, or rules. Often I had to wait for a single mistake to capitalize on. Today, if you win two of three rounds—even if your opponent finishes the round choking you—you're saved by the bell, and you win because you won the previous two. Don't get me wrong: the tough guys are still tough, and the warrior spirit is still there, and the chance of major injuries, especially brain injuries, is even greater now.

The modern MMA fighters are training like killing machines, and the divisions between strikers and ground fighters are not as great as they once were. Everyone is pretty skilled at everything now. Strikers can fight on the ground well enough to get back up, and ground fighters can strike well enough to punch their way into a clinch and take the fight to the ground. Today, some think that if you win without getting stitches or two black eyes, you're cheating. I do not share this view.

DEVASTATION

MY CHILDREN WERE GROWING UP QUICKLY. ALTHOUGH THEY ALL trained with me, they were also discovering passions of their own. By 1999, my younger son, Kron, was eleven. He was a natural at Jiu Jitsu but was more interested in skateboarding. Kaulin was now thirteen, an excellent all-around athlete emerging as a natural leader at school and in team sports. Kauan was fifteen and still in love with dancing and music. The girls loved to train Jiu Jitsu with me, but they weren't interested in competing. I never pushed them; they had other interests, and I respected and supported them in whatever direction they wanted to go.

I always tried to be present in my girls' lives. I gave them love, support, and advice on and off the mats, but I have to be honest, this was much harder for me to do with them than with my boys. I respected their accomplishments and supported them with the best teachers and schools that I could find, but they were on such a different path from the one that I had followed. My girls went to the best private schools in LA. I knew nothing about chemistry, modern art, or ballet. Their classmates were the children of some of the most powerful people in America. If Kauan needed help with a piano arrangement, I couldn't help her the same way I could help the boys. It was so different from preparing Rockson or Kron for a Jiu Jitsu tournament. I definitely rejected my dad's view that women belonged in the kitchen and the nursery. I wanted my girls to be strong and go in any direction they chose, and they were well on their way.

My older son, Rockson, was seventeen and devoted to Jiu Jitsu and his quest to become the greatest Gracie of his generation. Like me, Rockson had little interest in school and spent most of his time training and teaching at our academy. I worried about him growing up in my shadow and having to live up to both my reputation and our family name. As Rockson got older, he grew even more reckless and would accept any challenge and fight anyone to prove himself. I was afraid that something bad was going to happen to him because his lack of concern for his physical safety had only gotten worse. During a Calvin Klein modeling job, he jumped from the roof of the house where they were shooting into the swimming pool and nearly killed himself. Another time, he wanted to get into a party that he was not invited to, so he took off his shirt, walked up to the giant bouncer, and asked him, "If I fight you and win, can I get into the party?" The bouncer was so shocked that he let him into the party . . . without a fight. There was little I could do to rein him in because Rockson was now making his own money teaching Jiu Jitsu and modeling.

With kids, you have to accept the fact that you are not in control of their outcomes. You plant the seeds and nurture them as best you can, but at a certain point, you have to let go. No matter how much knowledge, love, money, or advice you give them, they will fly once their own wings are strong enough. Then they will chart their own courses through life. A father must accept his children for who they are, not who he would like them to be.

In November 1999, I returned to Tokyo with Rockson and Kim to corner for my brother Royler in a fight against veteran Japanese wrestler Kazushi Sakuraba. He was much bigger than my brother and had already had some MMA success against Jiu Jitsu fighters who were not members of my family. Victory was by submission only and the referee was not allowed to stop the fight. When the match began, Royler was unable to take Sakuraba to the ground, and the Japanese fighter methodically kicked my brother's legs until they were bruised. Thirteen minutes in, Sakuraba caught Royler in a kimura, and even though he didn't tap, the referee stopped the fight before the round ended. Because the rules stated clearly that the fight could not end by referee interference, there were some harsh words between our camp and the promoters. Then Sakuraba grabbed the microphone and challenged me to fight. The crowd went wild.

That night, someone knocked on Rockson's hotel door and when he opened it five big Japanese guys were standing in front of him. "Where is Rickson?" one asked.

"No, he's not in this room," Rockson said, then slammed the door shut and called my phone. "Fuck! Some yakuza guys are here looking for you!" The thugs never came to my door.

The Japanese fans still liked me, but the promoters were determined to find a Japanese fighter who could beat me. Even when I was fighting a Japanese fighter, many of the fans rooted for me because they felt that I represented their values better than some of my opponents. My relationship with the Japanese fans transcended flags and nationalities. I felt I had been adopted by the Japanese because I was a living reference to what by the 1990s were the lost ways of the Bushido code. While this bond with Japanese people was wonderful and affirming, it was not exactly what the promoters had in mind.

After Royler's fight, Kim negotiated the terms of my next fight, and I signed the contract. After some tense negotiations, the Japanese agreed to pay me $1.5 million if I won. The promoters didn't want me to fight a journeyman like Sakuraba. Instead they wanted me to fight Masakatsu Funaki, their biggest MMA star. Unlike Takada, Funaki was an extremely experienced fighter who had beaten some of the biggest names among the early MMA: Ken Shamrock, Frank Shamrock, Bas Rutten, and many others. Ten years younger than me and forty pounds heavier, Funaki was not just a pro wrestler. The promoters had picked the Japanese fighter who had the best chance of beating me. Funaki later said that when he was offered the fight he considered it *kakutougi*, "combat." In traditional *kakutougi*, if you lose, you die. I knew that Funaki, like me, was never going to tap.

Six months later, I was back in Japan. This time my body felt good—my back had healed—and I was ready. After my fight camp in the mountains, we traveled to Tokyo for the fight. It was the main event of Colosseum 2000, which forty thousand people attended and another thirty million watched on pay-per-view. The second Funaki stepped out from behind the curtain in the Tokyo Dome and stood at the top of a long staircase clad in a navy blue samurai kimono with a sword on his belt, the crowd roared. He made his way to the ring with Takada in tow and reaching it, he held up his sword, said a short prayer, touched the blade to his forehead, and then stepped into the ring. Unlike some of the fighters I faced in Japan, this opponent had no palpable fear. He was totally focused on defeating me.

The fight started and I came in for the clinch, but Funaki hit me with an overhand right. We wound up in the corner, trading tit-for-tat punches and knees. Nine minutes into the fight, Funaki grabbed my neck and attempted a guillotine choke. I was able to drag him to the ground, but he hit me in the eye on the way down. By the time we landed on the canvas, I had no vision, because the blow broke the orbital bones in my eye socket. My mind was still working properly and none of my internal gauges were redlining, so I felt I could still manage the situation. If anything, I embraced this as an opportunity to show that my decades-long winning streak was not a fluke but a result of training and methodology. I knew the only way Funaki could beat me was by knocking me out. If today was to be my last day, so be it. I would not cry, beg, or sell my soul to survive.

Funaki jumped to his feet and started kicking my legs. When I made no effort to get up, the crowd realized that I was hurt. The Japanese fans cheered every time he kicked my legs. Even though Royler was screaming, "Stand up! Stand up!" I took my time, breathed, and regrouped while everything boiled around me. I absorbed the kicks and tried not to touch my eye, so that my opponent wouldn't realize how badly I was hurt. I let Funaki kick my legs, hoping that my vision would return. When it did not, I resigned myself to fighting him blind.

Although he kicked me more than thirty times, he never went for the kill when he had me in the crosshairs, and that was his mistake. Shortly after I accepted my blindness, some vision returned to one eye. I landed a kick to Funaki's knee that gave me the distance to stand up safely. I sensed that he was trying to rest, so I attacked with total commitment, and took him back down to the mat. Once I had him on his back, he did not quit despite there being no escape. Funaki was a true warrior! I punched him in the face more than twenty times before he turned his back. Even as I was choking him unconscious, he never tapped, but he went to sleep.

Funaki later said that by refusing to tap, he was accepting his own death and was willing to die rather than surrender. He said that when I got him in the choke at the end of the fight, he thought he was going to die because he hadn't given his cornermen a towel to throw into the ring. The referee didn't stop me, I stopped myself. When Funaki came back to his senses, he later said that he was filled with joy because he was still alive. In his mind, because I released the choke, he got a second chance to live.

My brother Royler, my sons Rockson and Kron, and the rest of my team jumped into the ring to celebrate what was an emotional win for all of us. This fight was the closest that anyone had ever come to beating me and we all knew it.

Immediately after our fight, an emotional Funaki apologized to his fans. He said that because he considered this fight *kakutougi*, not a sport, there were no second chances, and he announced his retirement. A year or so later, I spoke to him. I had been concerned about Funaki and how he would recover from the defeat and get on with his life. I was relieved when he thanked me and told me that our fight was one of the greatest experiences in his life because it changed his perspective and made him reevaluate many things. When he told me how honored he was to fight me, I told him that the honor was mine. Anyone who was deadly serious about his mission and prepared to sacrifice his life for it had my utmost respect. Now the Japanese promoters were eager to pit me against Kazushi Sakuraba, who had beaten my brother Royler, but I was not prepared to commit to another fight until my eye was fully healed, so during the fall of 2000, I traveled to Brazil.

Earlier that year, Rockson had injured his knee while training. It was slow to heal, and I think he felt his dream of becoming a champion fighter was slipping away. While I was in Rio, there were rumors going around that Rockson was a prospective member in an LA street gang. His fascination and association with the gangs set him on narrow path that had nothing to do with the one that I tried to lead him down to make him a great Gracie fighter.

By the time I returned to Los Angeles, Rockson was getting ready to leave for New York with his Brazilian girlfriend. I was worried because he was going behind enemy lines. Throughout the 1990s, East Coast and West Coast rappers were at war. Rockson's hatred for everything East Coast— clothes, music, culture, even the pizza—was tribal. *Why was he going there now?* I asked myself. A friend who knew my son well warned me earlier in the year that if he stayed on his present path, it would not end well. Now his words rang in my ears.

After Rockson left for the East Coast, I received a message from him that he had made it to New York and that everything was going well. When we didn't hear from him for over a month, I wasn't that worried, because he was still using his ATM card in New York City. A month later, December had turned to January, and we still had not heard from him. Now I was truly worried. My cousin Renzo's academy was in New York City, and some of his students were policemen, so I asked Renzo if he would try to find my son. A few days later, a shaken Renzo called and told me that an officer had found a photograph of an unidentified corpse at the coroner's office with a tattoo that read RICKSON GRACIE #1 DAD.

Up to this point, Rockson had been a missing person. This was the confirmation that he was gone. After I hung up the phone, the whole family melted into tears. Kim, seated beside me, looked hopeless. I told the kids that Rockson had moved on to another life and was now with Rolls. Now, representing the Gracie family, I had to go to New York City for the physical confirmation. I knew in my heart that my son was dead.

Twenty-four hours later, I was in New York. Renzo didn't have to say anything when I met him; I could tell by the look on his face that it was true. He introduced me to the policeman, who showed me a postmortem photograph of Rockson. After I confirmed that it was my son, he told me that Rockson was buried at a place called Potter's Field, a graveyard for New York City's unknown dead. I was numb with shock when I learned that he had died alone and that his unidentified body was buried in a pauper's grave.

I flew back to Los Angeles and when I walked into our house in the Palisades with my son's ashes in my backpack, the finality of the situation hit me. Despite my best efforts to remain strong, I broke down and cried with my family. I cried for days.

We held Rockson's memorial service at the Self-Realization Fellowship center on Sunset Boulevard. It was a beautiful event, attended by hundreds, and we were moved by the outpouring of support from friends, family, and students. I tried to remain strong, but the truth was that the grief was much more powerful than I was. I played the role of the unflappable stoic warrior, but inside I was destroyed yet thought I couldn't show this wound in front of my friends and family. It took a long time for me to realize how deep this pain was and that I had to surrender to it and accept it in order to be reborn as a different person. The grief of losing a family member, especially one's child, is beyond anything I could have ever imagined.

About three weeks after Rockson's passing, the Japanese offered me $5 million to fight Sakuraba. This certainly would have been the most important fight of my career. The proposed terms were unprecedented at that time in MMA. But when they offered it to me, I was still trying to figure out what had happened to my son. I wanted to find out what had happened but do so out of the public eye, so I told people that he'd died in a motorcycle accident to buy time while I looked into the strange circumstances of his death. There were many things that didn't make sense. I didn't care about money or fame or notoriety at that time; I just wanted to discover the truth—for me and my family.

We eventually learned that Rockson died of an unusual drug overdose in December and his body was found in the Providence Hotel, a $10-a-night skid row hotel on the Bowery. According to the medical examiner's report, he died from an overdose of cocaine, opiates, sleeping pills, and an antihistamine. Why would he have taken such a lethal combination of drugs? Why was Rockson in a hotel full of homeless men and drug dealers? I asked myself these questions, but they were impossible to process.

Unbeknownst to me, at roughly the same time, a friend and student who lived in New York City and had known Rockson since he was a boy began looking into the case. He was a private investigator with a high-level contact in the New York Police Department and in the city's Chinatown. This was significant because the Providence Hotel was right on the border of Chinatown. After visiting the hotel, my friend believed that he could find out what happened. When he asked me if I would like him to reach out to his associates for help, I told him that I appreciated his efforts but asked him to stop investigating the matter. No act of vengeance or justice was going to bring my son back.

I didn't tell my friend that I already knew Rockson had been murdered. Roughly a month after his death, someone sent his suitcase back to our house. Inside it was a hand-drawn picture of the Grim Reaper standing on a mound of skulls. I immediately recognized this gesture as a demonstration of power fueled by hatred. I raised my kids to be responsible, in charge, to make good decisions under pressure, and to rise above whatever fray they were in. Rockson chose a different and more dangerous path, and this was the end that I had long been dreading.

When I found out the truth about my son's passing, I made an unequivocal decision to walk away from the Sakuraba fight. Regrouping my family and helping them heal was more important to me than anything else. I had lived the Gracie ideology of toughness, stoicism, and grace under pressure my entire life, but after Rockson died, I don't know if it failed me as much as I abandoned it. I could have brought all of my warrior values to bear so as to stay on my feet, but my family could not. I could have tried to keep myself from crying like a child. I could have said things like "God knows what he's doing" or scheduled my next fight and taken my pain out on Sakuraba. I could have numbed myself with drugs and alcohol.

I felt that by suppressing my emotions, I would be creating a mask that might make me look strong but would have just made me numb inside. Instead I thought that it was important to be fragile and let myself feel whatever pain, doubt, loss, weakness, and emptiness I needed to feel, to be honest enough to say, "Fuck! I don't know what to do."

My most important responsibility was to my family. They needed all of me and I would never get a second chance to help them. It was never even a choice. Although our marriage had been strained for many years, Kim and I came together with love and acceptance for each other in the aftermath of Rockson's death. We put our differences aside and focused on our children.

My father and I also reconciled. When Hélio and I met in Los Angeles, he told me that I had to accept Rockson's loss, and he comforted me through the never-ending process. My father believed in reincarnation. He thought that death was not the end, but rather a passage to another existence where my brother Rolls, and now Rockson, would be waiting for us.

At first, I felt that I could rationalize this tragedy and move forward with my life, but then I realized that rationality cannot always suppress raw emotion. I went deep into the hole of grief, hit the bottom, and stayed there for almost three years. I just obeyed my heart and accepted the fact that my life would never be the same after losing my son. I had no idea what the future held, and I no longer cared. Sadness was a big part of my new life, from which I thought I would never recover.

I allowed myself to feel and absorb the trauma. I stopped surfing, teaching, training, and exercising; none of it brought me any pleasure. I just stayed at home, took my kids to school, and talked and cried with them about Rockson.

When you talk about loss, there are so many clichés—about strength, perseverance, prayer, friends, family, the future. None of them mattered. I'd been tied to a three-hundred-pound rock and dumped into the sea. When I hit the bottom, I had to decide, deep down, whether I would come back to the surface or not.

One day I was walking on the hillside above our house and decided to climb a tree. When I got to the top, I could see the ocean, and I visualized the past, present, and future together with my late son. "Wherever you are, Rockson," I said to the great wide world, "we are at peace, we are connected, and eventually we will be together again." At that moment, I decided to build a wooden platform where I could meditate and talk to Rockson whenever I wanted. As soon as I got the idea, I felt inspired for the first time since his passing. I would build a monument to him with my own hands that would express my love and be a gift to his everlasting spirit.

I went to the hardware store, got all of the supplies I needed, and for weeks spent most of my time in the tree. I would come down in the evening to shower, eat, and sleep, but I would be back at it the next day.

While I was building the platform, a blue jay kept coming around to check out what I was doing. In the beginning, he just watched me intently. He was probably on his guard because I had come into his territory so suddenly. But as time went on, he would venture closer and closer. As a sign of respect, I made him an offering of peanuts each day. I rolled the peanuts to him on the wooden floor of the platform, and he would come closer and start to eat them. As the days passed, the blue jay got more and more curious and we grew more comfortable with each other. The distance between us kept shrinking and shrinking, until one day I held out a peanut and he hopped into my hand to eat it. After that, I could just make a clicking sound with my mouth, and he would fly over to me.

Blue jays are wise and noble birds. They are curious but can also be fearlessly aggressive and have been known to attack owls and even hawks. They also form monogamous pairs for life. Once the birds mate, they protect their family until the end.

Sometime after he began flying into my hand, he and his mate built a nest right above our front door, and I watched them raise their offspring. The blue jays were now part of my family, and I was part of theirs.

After I varnished the platform, I hung up a laminated photo of Rockson that I could look at while I prayed and meditated. I felt happier and lighter but still not fully recovered. I wanted to let go of the rock of grief that I was holding, but I couldn't. With my work on the platform, I had given something with all of my heart to Rockson, but now I had to let him go. Many days, I would go to the platform, light incense, and meditate. I had done my penance and now I wanted to find happiness.

One day I remembered something that my dad always used to say: "Nothing can be a hundred percent positive or a hundred percent negative." I spent a long time trying to find something positive that I could take away from this tragedy. After much meditation, I realized that I had never really valued time. I thought that I controlled time and could put things off, like talking to my son, until later. After Rockson's departure, I understood that there is no tomorrow, because life can change forever in the blink of an eye. I needed to do my best every day because it might be my last. I no longer had the luxury of wasted time!

Rockson's death affected everyone in my family differently. My daughter Kauan was inspired to study dance and went on to earn a college degree in it. More important, dance gave her an outlet for her grief and a way to find herself. Kau-an's final project for her degree was a performance that she choreographed as a memorial for her late brother. It brought us all to tears.

My younger daughter, Kaulin, continued to excel in sports and considered playing college volleyball at one point. She was a born leader. What impressed me most about Kaulin was that she was not afraid to go after the things she wanted in life. When she decided that she wanted to go to a very exclusive private school for girls or a college in Switzerland, she got the applications, filled them out, and pursued her objectives with relentless, single-minded determination.

Losing Rockson put Kron on the path to martial-arts greatness. On some level, I think Rockson knew that Kron had the natural talent and the tools to be even better than he. Like all of my kids, he had trained all his life but was never as interested in Jiu Jitsu as Rockson. Now it was his turn to shine. Kron had always been a great observer. The youngest child sees everybody in the family for who they are and then decides who he is going to be. Even as a child, he had a great deal of sensitivity and natural intuition. Unlike Rockson, who wanted only me as his point of reference, Kron had three important women in his life: his mother and two sisters. They gave him a different perspective and a much better understanding of emotion than I had at his age. This natural intuition helped him in Jiu Jitsu because it enhanced his ability to respond spontaneously to his opponent. He learned quickly how to read his opponents and how to remain one step ahead of them.

Even though they were brothers, Rockson and Kron were completely different. Rockson was emotional, intense, and intent on proving himself a Gracie warrior. Kron was much more observant, analytical, and calm. He wanted to do things right and always be at his best. In one of their last conversations, Rockson told Kron that he was a Gracie and to give 110 percent, and never quit in whatever it was that he chose to do. After Rockson died, Kron took that to heart and was now on a mission to become the next apex predator in the Gracie food chain.

In his effort to honor Rockson, he took on a huge responsibility and connected with me and our family traditions in a way that he hadn't in the past. Kron's calm demeanor allowed him to do many things that his brother was unable to do. He trained hard and followed the Gracie protocols. He also impressed me by asking intelligent questions about the things that would soon be his daily bread, like pressure, fear, and courage.

Kron gathered all of the information he needed to become a champion and analyzed it in a way that would serve his ends. In an effort to fulfill his destiny, he wanted to know everything Rockson thought, everything I thought, and everything Hélio thought before interpreting this body of knowledge. Kron was trying to gather all of the mental, spiritual, and physical elements that he would need to succeed.

The more Kron won, the less attached he became to winning. After he realized that the outcome of a fight does not define you as a person, he improved by leaps and bounds. He trained as hard as humanly possible, and when he competed, he let the chips fall where they might. Win, lose, or draw, he would be back in the academy on Monday and train as if the fight had never happened. Like me, Kron never fought for points, advantages, or judges' decisions; he always went for the kill. As a purple and brown belt, he won fifty-one straight matches by submission. After every fight, he would open his gi and kiss the image of Rockson that he had sewn inside. He lost his first match as a black belt, but went on to win every title there was to win in Jiu Jitsu before going on to fight MMA.

When my father died in his sleep in 2009 at the age of ninety-five, I was in Europe with Kron for the European Jiu Jitsu Championship. We received the news the day of the tournament and knew that we could not go back to Brazil for the funeral. Instead we went back to our hotel room and held our own memorial. We cried and shared memories.

The day Hélio died, Kron represented his grandfather on the mat as Hélio would have liked. He won both of his matches by submission, and after he won the European title, he kissed the picture of Rockson as always and bowed to the giant mural of Hélio the tournament organizers put up to commemorate his life. It was a beautiful moment for both of us. Hélio and Carlos Gracie's legacies were now being carried and upheld by a third generation.

By the time my dad died, he and I had put all of the bad feelings over the UFC behind us and reconciled our differences. We still had a great deal of mutual respect and love for each other, and we became father and son again. Even as he got old and his memory about day-to-day things began to fade, Hélio's memories of his fights, the crazy horses he rode, and his love affairs with vicious dogs all remained vivid. When my father looked at me, there was always a twinkle in his eye. He never stopped being proud of me as a fighter, a champion, and above all, a representative of the Gracie family. After I retired, he still considered me the champ. "How are you feeling? How has the training been going?" he would ask. "Nobody can kick your ass!"

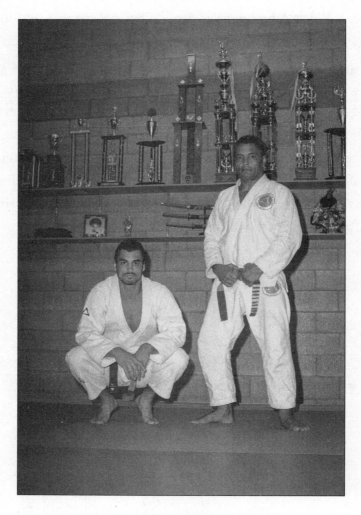

KRON AND RICKSON GRACIE.
PHOTOGRAPH COURTESY OF STEFAN KOCEV.

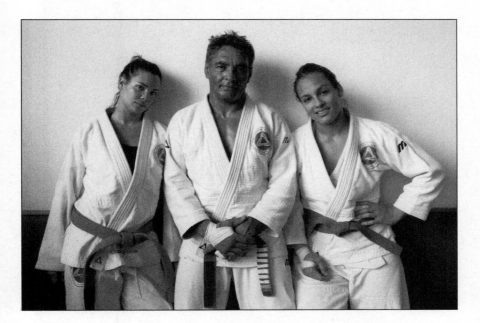

KAUAN, RICKSON, AND KAULIN GRACIE, RIO, 2014.
PHOTOGRAPH COURTESY OF STEFAN KOCEV.

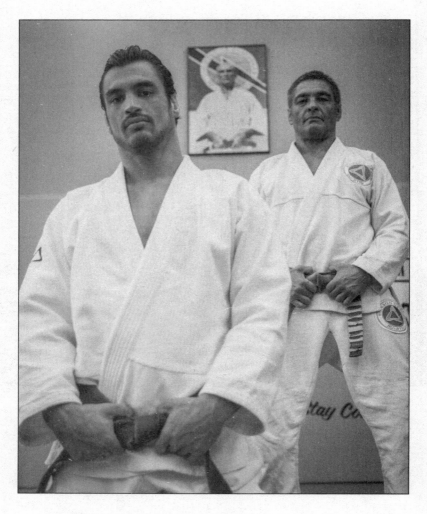

KRON AND RICKSON GRACIE WITH A PORTRAIT OF HÉLIO.
PHOTOGRAPH COURTESY OF STEFAN KOCEV.

REBIRTH

I SPENT FIVE YEARS REBUILDING MYSELF AND MY FAMILY, WORK-ing through the grief of losing my son. Our recovery was more emotional and spiritual than rational or intellectual. Looking back on the experience, I can now see that a part of me died and I was reborn as a different person with a greater appreciation for how precious and fragile life is. During the years I spent grieving and rebuilding, I searched for a reason to be happy again and found three: my children, my family, and Jiu Jitsu.

When it comes to my heart, I am always very honest with myself. Even though I had a nice house, a wonderful family, great friends, devoted students, a thriving academy, and a new truck with new surfboards on the roof, I was unhappy and uninspired. One morning I woke up in our big, empty house and asked myself, "What am I doing here?"

After Rockson's death, Kim and I had come together to manage the crisis and had raised three children who developed strong wings and were taking off in their own directions. Kauan was living in Italy, Kron was running the academy, and Kaulin was attending college. I had been so focused on getting everyone else through this tragedy that I had not attended to myself and had just been surviving, not living. Likewise, Kim was also just managing this crisis.

Happiness is not a static thing. You have to work at it by confronting and overcoming challenges.

After all that Kim and I had been through, I didn't want to lie to her or cheat on her. More than anything else, I just wanted to go home. Yes, Brazil is Brazil, and with it comes traffic, crime, and corruption. But Brazil is home. I needed the friends, the food, and the passion that, to me, represent it.

I called Kim into the living room and told her I wanted a divorce. She was shocked and asked me how I planned to do it. "It's simple," I said. "You can have everything."

And that is what happened. Before I left, we finalized our divorce, and I signed over the house in Pacific Palisades, the farm in Brazil, and the apartment in Rio to Kim. My sudden decision to get a divorce and move back to Rio was difficult for my kids, because they felt that I had abandoned them and their mother. While I understood their perspective, I had to figure out what I wanted to do with the rest of my life.

When I moved back to Rio, I made one vow to myself: after years of paying private-school tuitions, mortgages, and car payments, I would now always make more money than I spent. It sounds basic, but it isn't in a world based on easy credit. If you make $1 million a month but spend $1.2 million, you'll never get your head above water. Even more important, if you base your life around money, it's easy to corner yourself. Say you want to live in Malibu, you'll need at least $3 million for a house, and that's just the beginning. Soon you'll want a Porsche, because all the neighbors have them. Then you'll want your kids to go to the best private school, because that's where their friends go. As your expectations continue to rise, slowly but surely, the things you own will own you. In a few years, you won't need to make $5 million a year; you'll need to make $10 million. When money becomes more important than happiness, your life passes you by, because you can't lower your guard and enjoy yourself. Money is a tricky thing: it can bring you freedom and happiness, but it can also bring pain and anxiety. I was now determined to find a healthy balance.

I felt like a tourist when I returned home, because so many things had changed. Most days, I would go to the beach in the morning to do my exercise routines and surf. After I finished surfing, I would sit in the sand and think about what I was going to do to fill up my days. Some days I thought about opening a snack stand on the beach and selling fish and beer. Other days I thought about opening a Jiu Jitsu academy or even fighting one last MMA bout. But when I really thought about it, I realized that I didn't want to run a small business or have an academy or fight again. These were just familiar routines that would fill my time, but they would not inspire or empower me. For me to get back to my best, my mind, heart, and spirit had to be in alignment.

I had always enjoyed giving seminars. I found them stimulating; you parachute into a foreign environment and have to quickly make sense of students you have never met. When I decided that I was going to start teaching seminars, I reached out to friends and students all over the world to set up them up. It was important to me not to do too many at first, so that I could give each one all of my energy and have enough time to recharge my batteries before the next one. But soon enough, I began to travel far and wide, from Europe to Australia, teaching students of all abilities from all walks of life.

One of the biggest challenges of seminars is managing egos. People communicate who they are, especially in the world of martial arts, by the way they present themselves to me. At each seminar, I do a quick survey of the students. Some are friendly because they are fans, while others are a bit more circumspect because they are curious but not yet convinced of Jiu Jitsu's efficacy. Then there are those who are slightly hostile because they have come to challenge me and hope to make a name for themselves by submitting me. The overwhelming majority of my students are incredibly gracious and grateful for the opportunity to learn. Those with humility and innocent curiosity are the easiest to teach, because their minds are open to new things. It is difficult to teach people to relearn things they have been doing wrong for decades. But if the spirit is willing, the mind and body will follow.

Sometimes, I can't be nice or gentle: I have to stretch an arm or squeeze a neck to make my point. Big egos and closed minds usually come hand in hand. Occasionally, a student's shell will be so hard that I have to crack it first in order to teach them. To do this, I have to show them—not tell them— what I am teaching them works.

I once gave a seminar in Alabama. Most of the students were wearing gis, but some wore shorts and T-shirts. Standing on the edge of the mat, looking at me like I owed him money, was a big guy dressed head-to-toe in camouflage. He gave me mean looks throughout the seminar and was not interested in learning Jiu Jitsu.

At the end of every seminar, I invite the students to spar with me. We start on our knees, and 95 percent of the matches are very friendly even if my opponents are competitive and trying their hardest to beat me. When camo man's turn to spar came, he stepped onto the mat and didn't even bother to take off his boots. I said "go" and he immediately attacked with all of his strength. I don't mind if people go hard, but when camo man began to scratch my face, he crossed a line. I try not to show anger in seminars because I don't want to poison the atmosphere by stooping down to the level of the lowest common denominator, but escalation comes with a price. I said nothing, as I took his arm and stretched it until he screamed.

Another time, I did a huge seminar in Paris for hundreds of students. Judo is extremely popular in France, and there were quite a few men in the room with bent noses and cauliflower ears who were very comfortable on the mat. Everyone was friendly and receptive to what I was teaching, except for one burly judoka who did not smile once in three hours. Normally, I spar with everyone, but I couldn't in this seminar because of the large number of people. Everyone raised their hands when I asked, "Who wants to spar?" I picked the thirty toughest-looking guys, including, of course, the big judoka, whom I saved for last. By the time I got to him, he was so eager for his match that he was on the mat before my last opponent had finished tapping. I baited him with an unbalanced throw, when he extended his arm to defend against it, I caught him in an armlock. After the big judoka tapped in less than ten seconds, he was furious. When he demanded to have another match, I told him to take a seat.

After the seminar ended and I was driving back to my hotel, my French manager turned to me and asked, "Rickson, how do you know how to pick the guys you pick?" "I can always smell tigers," I replied, "no matter how hard they try to hide their stripes." The Frenchman laughed and then he told me that the big judoka was an Olympian who had spent the past year boasting about how ineffective Jiu Jitsu would be against him. In life, there will always be people like the big judoka, and it is important not to respond to their egotism and arrogance with egotism and arrogance. I did not engage in the way that he expected, so I defined the terms of the conflict and beat him easily.

For me as a teacher, seminars are both exhausting and exhilarating. Many people can teach armlocks and chokes, but I approach teaching in a much more holistic manner. In order to learn my Jiu Jitsu, you have to *feel* it. That is why I call my practice "invisible Jiu Jitsu." I believe that only when students feel things like base and connection can they understand them. Without this tactile knowledge and mastery of the basics, a student can learn every technique in the world but still not understand the essence of Jiu Jitsu. For example, many students have been doing the *upa* (neck-bridge escape) wrong for decades. After I show them where they are going wrong and make some tiny adjustments, they leave with a new weapon in their arsenal and a sense of power they didn't have before they met me. This is extremely gratifying for me as a teacher.

As rewarding as the seminars were for me, I did not like what I saw when I dove headfirst back into the world of Jiu Jitsu. Competition and the need to play within its rules had transformed our martial art into a sport and a game. A top Jiu Jitsu competitor might have five tough bouts in a single day. Why would he go all out and exhaust himself in his first match when he could get ahead on points and then stall and run out the clock? Many modern competitors adopt smart strategies that minimize their risks and maximize their competitive rewards. They become experts at holding advantageous positions, but the fluid movement, the improvisational back-and-forth exchanges—like the ones Rolls and I used to have—are a fraction of what they once were and should be. For this reason, I was proud of Kron, probably in the same way my father was proud of me, for winning all of his important Jiu Jitsu titles by submission, never by points.

I had plenty of time in Brazil between seminars to think about how to bring the community closer together. While I respected the top Jiu Jitsu competitors as remarkable athletes, I did not consider them complete martial artists, because they ignored the self-defense aspect of the practice. Fights in real life are unpredictable, and often your only goal is survival.

If a mob turns on you, it doesn't matter who you are—me, US Navy SEAL Jocko Willink, Mark Kerr, anyone—your only option is a strategic retreat. I experienced a situation like this when I was seventeen and in the south of Brazil for Carnival. We were standing in front of a nightclub talking to some girls, and a guy sucker-punched me. After I hit him back, the whole neighborhood attacked me. Suddenly twenty guys were chasing me down the street. Somebody in the mob threw a big piece of wood at my head. I managed to get my arm up in time to deflect it, but I also realized that if I made one mistake, I would be in deep trouble. I just kept running and fighting, running and fighting, until finally the mob got tired and gave up. Although I used very little actual Jiu Jitsu, my martial arts mind-set was the thing that saved me. I don't care if a student is only interested in the sport of Jiu Jitsu; every blue belt needs to know how to block a punch, clinch, take someone to the ground and control them. Even more important, they need to know how to use the guard to defend against punches and head butts in the event of a real-life assault.

For the first time in many years, I felt a renewed sense of purpose. Now I wanted everything in my life—a conversation with a stranger, a new project, or a Jiu Jitsu seminar—to have meaning. I refused to waste time on things that I did not value, and I left other people's expectations behind.

After just a few seminars, I bought a cheap car and moved into an apartment near the beach. Because I was spending only 5 percent of what I made, I was soon able to make a down payment on a small house near my favorite beach. I was beginning to feel good again.

One night, I went to a Santana concert in Rio with a friend and saw an attractive woman holding a motorcycle helmet standing nearby. I did not approach her, but we made eye contact and she smiled at me. After the concert ended, I went down to Ipanema Beach to eat pizza at one of my favorite restaurants and whom do I see but the woman who smiled at me at the concert, eating with her family.

I don't believe in coincidences—so I approached her and introduced myself. Her name was Cassia, and she was a university student. After we finished eating, I took Cassia and her family to my friend's nightclub. We spent the night dancing together and went to the beach the next day. We tried to keep things casual, so that each of us had the freedom to pursue our careers, but we swiftly fell in love.

When I moved into Cassia's apartment, I was utterly focused on our relationship, since I no longer wanted to waste time and energy. Cassia is an independent woman who has her own career and aspirations, and we are often apart. Infidelity, jealousy, doubt—these are never issues for us. After meeting Cassia, I was happy for the first time in many years, and this played a big role in inspiring me to reinvent Jiu Jitsu.

My overhead was so low in Brazil that one seminar paid my living expenses for six months. This left me plenty of time to think about how I could improve Jiu Jitsu. Initially, I dreamed of unifying the Jiu Jitsu community, and to achieve that goal, I formed the Jiu Jitsu Global Federation. In retrospect, I was very idealistic. I was careful to be inclusive and put together a commission composed of Jiu Jitsu's greatest practitioners, teachers, and elder statesmen to help guide us. I was sure that, if nothing else, we could come up with better rules for the tournaments, standardize techniques and belts testing, and do other practical things to help consolidate and legitimate our martial art.

I decided that the best place to launch the Jiu Jitsu Global Federation was in America, so I moved back to the United States with Cassia in 2012 after we got married. After Cassia spent time in the US with me, she was impressed by how well things functioned and what a civil society it was compared to her homeland. It was a difficult time in Brazil, wherein the violence and chaos seemed to be getting worse with every passing year. We both wanted to move to America and found a house in Palos Verdes.

In the fall of 2013, I called my most trusted black-belt teachers and students to attend a closed-door, two-day meeting in Redondo Beach. After we enjoyed a nice dinner and reunion, I whistled, called the meeting to order, and spoke to them from my heart. "Our culture, the culture of Jiu Jitsu, is under siege," I explained. "We have become the minority and our style is dying! Our system was designed for the weak to defend themselves against the strong. The guy with genetic gifts is not the one we developed it for. Pretty medals and fancy somersaults have no relationship to real life. If you don't know self-defense, you don't know Jiu Jitsu. You have to be ready to defend yourself from a punch, a headlock, or a bear hug. If you can't do that, you're just a tough guy with big ears and a good grip who's depending on physicality for success. This is not Gracie Jiu Jitsu!"

We spent the next two days reviewing self-defense techniques and discussing how we could restore Jiu Jitsu's effectiveness as a martial art. Although we got off to a good start and got a great deal of positive press, egos and vested interests soon began to get in the way. It got harder and harder to define—much less reach—a common goal. One problem was that Jiu Jitsu had split into different factions that did not communicate, much less train with one another. In the old days, a Jiu Jitsu fighter was prepared to compete with or without a gi and also fight *vale tudo* or MMA. In the modern world of Jiu Jitsu, many gi and no-gi fighters only grappled

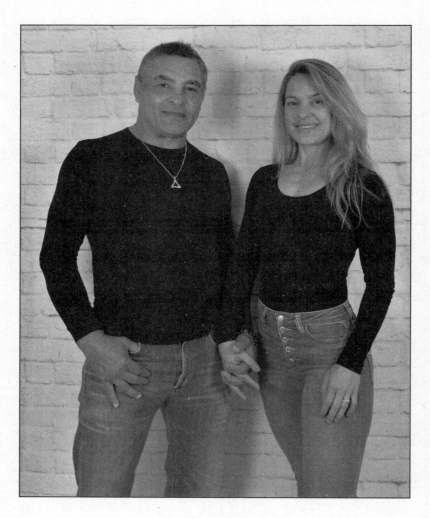

RICKSON WITH CASSIA.

PHOTO COURTESY OF CASSIA GRACIE.

and ruled out fighting *vale tudo* or MMA. Self-defense was meaningless to them because it wouldn't help them win tournaments. The biggest problem, however, was that people were making too much money off Jiu Jitsu to want to rock the boat.

After I faced the fact that I was not going to be the one to unify Jiu Jitsu, I realized that the most valuable thing I had was my knowledge and experience. I began to alter my vision, because I was much more interested in being of service to people than political infighting. More than anything else, I wanted to promote something that could be positive and beneficial for others—something I could be proud of. Once I made the commitment to be of service, things began to fall into place organically, because it coincided with my own life cycle.

As I approached the age of sixty, a lifetime's worth of extreme wear and tear on my body began to catch up with me. In addition to herniated disks in my back and neck, as well as shoulder problems, my hip was completely worn out and needed to be replaced. I tried to be stoic and will myself through the pain, but walking—never mind practicing Jiu Jitsu—was becoming more and more difficult.

After my hip-replacement operation, I embraced the process of recovery and rehabilitation and made physical therapy my full-time job. For someone my age, I recovered quickly and was back on the mat in no time. I believe the reason was not only because of my doctor or physical therapist, but also because of the mind-set and habits I had acquired from my lifetime of practicing martial arts. This experience made me realize that Jiu Jitsu needed to be accessible not just to athletes and fighters, but to everyone.

Up to this point, most of my students had been elite athletes—the tip of the spear, the top of the food chain. The aging process has made me realize how difficult it would be for a small, unathletic, insecure beginner—the very person Gracie Jiu Jitsu was invented for—to walk into one of today's academies and begin training. Getting big cauliflower ears, being in constant pain, having big guys in stinky gis sit on your face—these should not be the prerequisites for learning Jiu Jitsu.

In the old days, my father made students take forty private lessons before they ever set foot in an open group class. Hélio believed that Jiu Jitsu was as much about building a student's confidence as it was about learning how to fight. The frustration, injuries, and egos that today's students encounter when they attempt to learn Jiu Jitsu will scare most people away. Even worse, it filters out those who need it most—the weak and insecure.

My goal today is to create a form of Jiu Jitsu that will empower the entire person, both on and off the mat. If I can make a nervous person feel more relaxed than they've ever felt before, I'm changing them from within in a way that a psychiatrist or a pill never can. Today, conflict comes in many forms, and physicality is only one aspect of it. Conflict follows humans wherever they go, and people adopt different strategies to cope with it. Modern enemies can strike in a text, an e-mail, or in a social media post. As the world of instant communications has evolved, many negative, unintended consequences have evolved with it. Fifty years ago, a ten-year-old boy went into his room only to sleep, because he spent all day outside playing. Today, if parents aren't careful, their children will spend the entire day alone in their rooms. We cannot dismiss technology, but why let it turn us into brains with vestigial bodies?

One of the worst side effects of technology is the way it has reduced direct human interaction. Because people can get almost everything they desire—food, entertainment, friendship, sex—via the screen, many have gotten to the point of being scared of face-to-face interaction. There are so many wonderful things that are impossible to experience on a screen: jumping into a cold river, making the drop on a big wave, and walking in the rain are just a few. Even worse, social media provides an arena for cowards to lurk in the cybershadows and say things that they would never dare say in person. Mike Tyson put it best when he said that social media has made people "way too comfortable with disrespecting people and not getting punched in the face for it."

Today I try to use Jiu Jitsu as a tool to teach patience, hope, strategy, emotional control, breathing, and many other things—all without conflict and competition. This allows those who need it most to learn the visible and invisible aspects of the art in ways that could help them in their everyday lives. I have developed a training routine wherein students learn and practice all of the movements and techniques of Jiu Jitsu in a cooperative instead of a competitive environment. I can teach the most critical invisible aspects of Jiu Jitsu, like base, timing, weight distribution, and connection, with little stress. In this type of class, I can have two beginners blocking punches and doing hip throws. Your training partner is there to help you, not fight you.

The idea of base is reflected in the triangle that is the symbol for Gracie Jiu Jitsu. If I push a ball, my energy will project and make it roll away. If I push a pyramid, it will stay rooted because of its powerful base. Even if I throw that pyramid, it always lands on a solid base. If my base is solid, I am ready to move and take any opportunity, either to deflect an opponent's energy or to use it against him. If I have both a base and a connection, my opponent will be forced to follow me like the tail of a comet.

I can incorporate martial-arts concepts into anyone's life and show them how to tap into their invisible power.

I believe that Jiu Jitsu is especially important for people today, because it forces them to connect with another human being. That is why I believe my most important mission is to use its practices to rehumanize people. Learning to breathe, physically connect, engage, detach, and disengage—these primal processes require people to trust their senses more than their thoughts, and in doing so reconnect them with their bodies.

If I walk into a room full of people, the first thing I do is connect with the energy in that room. I might sense happiness, envy, anger, admiration, innocence, love, naïveté—whatever is in that room I will capture if I allow my senses to do their jobs. Today, I live my life based on how I connect with the people and the environment around me. It usually starts with a question: "Why am I doing this? Is this worth my energy?" If my response is anything but positive, I disconnect, disengage, and go home to feed the animals in my yard or walk my dogs.

When we moved into our house in Palos Verdes, I went out of my way to make the neighborhood animals feel comfortable in our yard. Within a few months, I had made friends with the squirrels, raccoons, crows, and blue jays (different ones this time). I had one enemy, though, a feral cat who was always trying to kill the birds. I did not like cats; I thought that they were selfish, sneaky, and vicious. At first, I'd try to squirt him with the hose to scare him away, but he was too smart for that. One winter, it had been cold and rainy for weeks, and Cassia saw that the cat was wet and miserable without shelter. She felt sorry for him, so she put our dog's traveling case outside to give him shelter from the rain, and he started sleeping in the carrier.

One day, we noticed that the cat could barely walk because one of his feet was badly injured. The next time he entered the carrier, I closed it and took him to the veterinarian, who told us he had gotten into a fight with a raccoon. After the vet treated him, I brought him home and cut a hole in the garage door so he could recover and heal indoors. Once the cat was better, and perhaps grateful for what we had done for him, he stopped bothering the birds. He became my best friend and changed my mind about cats. We named him Ginger.

My cat reinforced my belief that the deeper my connections are, the more fulfilling my life becomes. The Japanese have an expression, *ichi-go ichi-e*, which roughly translates to "once in a lifetime." It could refer to a gathering of friends, a special meal, an epic day of surf, but the idea is to savor that occasion, because it will never come again. I share this view and believe that if you see every moment in life as a unique opportunity, you live with much more intensity and precision because you are using 100 percent of your energy, your voice, and your senses. It is always important to remember that. For example, if I were driving to the airport to fly to Japan and my daughter Kauan called and said, "Dad! I need to talk to you!" the old Rickson would have said, "Honey, I'll call you once I land in Japan." Today, I would pull over, park the car, and give her as much time as she needed. What if I miss the plane? Fuck the plane! There is always another flight, but I don't want to ever regret not taking my daughter's call.

I still love going to Japan, and not just for the business opportunities, but because I connected so deeply to the country and its culture during my years as a fighter. Many great fighters have fought in Japan, but few formed a bond with the Japanese people like mine. Even today, when I go there, people will bring their babies to my public events and ask me to put my hand on their heads. One time, I called

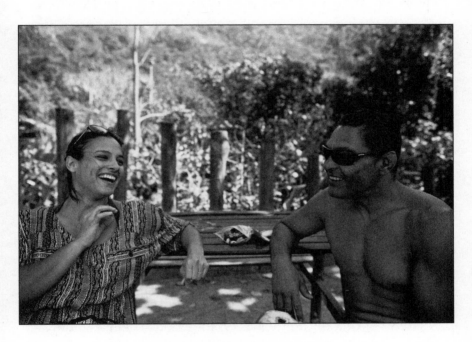

KAULIN AND RICKSON GRACIE, 2014.
PHOTOGRAPH COURTESY OF STEFAN KOCEV.

on a journalist from one of the nation's biggest magazines at a press conference. "Mister Gracie, I have just one question for you," he said. "How would you fight a polar bear?" I didn't laugh but really thought about it for a moment before replying.

"That's a good question," I said. "I have no intention to fight a polar bear and haven't thought of a strategy for that. But one thing is for sure! By the end of the fight, I'm going to have a nice fur coat, lots of meat, and a bear-teeth necklace!"

The last time I was in Japan, I was invited to go on a TV game show. The format of the show was simple: a doctor would press a pressure point on your foot, and if you could last thirty seconds, you win. Nobody had ever won before. When I got to the hotel where they were filming it, the cameras were set up and the doctor was already there. He was a short guy with giant forearms and short, thick fingers. I asked for a few minutes to prepare myself. When I did my breathing routine to put myself into fighting mode, I immediately felt that my honor was on the line. If I get caught in a joint lock in a real fight, even if it breaks my arm or ankle, I won't tap. Giving up or quitting is just not in my vocabulary. But the idea of being on TV, in front of millions of people, added even more pressure.

When the producer said "Go!" I thought to myself, *Cut my foot off and take it home, motherfucker! Take it, motherfucker! Take it!* Before I knew it, a bell rang, and the thirty seconds were up. The doctor was impressed and began doubting that he got the right pressure point because I didn't make a single sound. When he asked me how I did it, I told him that I focused as if I was in a fight, because I would never quit in a fight. I said, "With all due respect, I didn't see you as a doctor. I saw you as my opponent in a fight. I was expecting pain and defeated the pain with my mind-set." Afterward, I went to stand up and could barely walk to the elevator. The mind has incredible potential, but you have to dig deep to discover it. I can resist any physical pain if there is a reason. This is the heritage of my martial arts training and fighting, but now it is part of my soul.

On my best day now, I'm only 5 percent of what I once was as a fighter. However, my invisible power transcends my physicality and will be a part of me until the day I die. That is why, for me, Jiu Jitsu is about much more than fighting. It is a tool to teach people about themselves. It is great to see it become so popular and provide lucrative businesses for so many, but this has nothing to do with what I teach. Of my students, 98 percent train two or three days a week trying to perfect basic techniques and then testing them on a level playing field. Helping my students try to become better people, not just smashing-machines, is what motivates me. Jiu Jitsu is my philosophy, my sacred honor, and my family tradition. It has made me strong enough to forgive and confident enough to fight for my beliefs.

EPILOGUE

RECONCILED WITH MY BROTHER RORION WHEN I MOVED BACK TO the US in 2012. After all that I had been through, I still missed him. We had shared so much during the course of our lives, and there is still nobody who can make me laugh like Rorion. Today we don't talk much about the politics of Jiu Jitsu or business, but we laugh about Hélio and his crazy dogs, how he used to ride his horse next to the train tracks with a baby on the saddle, and the good times we spent with our extended family at Teresópolis. I love my brother, but people don't change. Rorion is still Rorion, and he sometimes acts as if I'm still a five-year-old he can hustle into shining his belt buckle and shoes.

In 2017, I was teaching a seminar in Las Vegas. As I was demonstrating a guard pass, there was some commotion in the back of the room that distracted my students. I tried to ignore it and keep teaching until I heard a very familiar voice say, "Are you sure, Rickson?" I looked up and saw my brother Rorion. Behind him stood my brother Royler, my cousins Jean Jacques and Carlos Machado, my old students Pedro Sauer, Carlos Valente, my dad's student Alvaro Barreto, and many other friends.

I was emotionally overwhelmed by this surprise and tried to gather my thoughts as Rorion began to talk to the crowd. "Since the explosion of Jiu Jitsu," he said, "people like Rickson are needed to teach classes and change peoples' lives all over the world." My mind was spinning trying to figure out what my brother had up his sleeve. This tribute was too unexpected and well executed for it to be genuine, right? "Once we found out that he was going to be in Las Vegas here," Rorion continued, "we decided that we should not wait any longer to give him his red belt."

Rorion pulled a red belt—the highest degree in Jiu Jitsu—out of his gi, hugged me and began to tie it around my waist.

I felt torn. While I was touched to see my friends and family and felt honored by the recognition, I knew that I was too young to wear a red belt. No matter what my accomplishments were, according to my family tradition, I have to be a black belt for forty years to be eligible to wear it. I whistled, asked everyone to sit down. "I'm not yet there," I explained.

"I don't want to be a special case; I want to be a regular one." Above all, I wanted to unify the community by following the rules like everyone else.

My brothers objected when I said that I would keep the red belt in my safe. Royler started to speak up, but Rorion cut him off and declared, "Because I said you're a red belt, you should wear a red belt. . . ." I knew that it was pointless to argue with Rorion, so I kissed both of my brothers and decided to just enjoy the moment with my family and friends. I wanted the message of the day—what all those present would remember—to be about the importance and power of a united Jiu Jitsu community.

I said, "The most important thing for us right now is to restore the traditions within Gracie Jiu Jitsu, introduce self-defense into every school, put the black belts at the service of the weaker ones, and ensure that the community benefits from people's ability to use martial arts in life." At this point, though, the tears came easier than the words. Whatever my principled objections to being awarded the red belt, I couldn't help but cry because I was overwhelmed by this show of love and support. I ended my speech quickly: "So, this is too tough for me now emotionally, and I have to digest this a little bit. Thank you."

After the seminar, I decided to put the red belt in my safe and not wear it again until I turn sixty-five. I can't tie a belt around my waist if I don't feel I deserve it. There is a reason the tradition asks that red belts be awarded after forty-five years: it is a recognition of wisdom earned over time and lifelong commitment to our art that transcends your victories in the ring.

I have fought my entire life, from pre-black-belt matches to challenge matches and in-house tournaments, from Jiu Jitsu to Sambo, from wrestling to *vale tudo*. When people ask me how many bouts I've fought, how do I count them? The number makes no difference to me. What matters is that I always led from the front lines and represented Jiu Jitsu with all of my heart. I may no longer fight, but I will always be a martial artist.

ACKNOWLEDGMENTS

FIRST, I WOULD LIKE TO THANK HÉLIO AND CARLOS GRACIE FOR creating our family's martial art. I would like to thank Orlando Cani for teaching me some of the most important lessons of my life. I want to thank my wife, Cassia, for her love and support. My brother Royler was one of my greatest supporters and will always hold a special place in my heart for that. My brother Rorion, despite our differences over the years, taught me how to teach and deserves a great deal of credit for the international success of Jiu Jitsu and MMA. I also want to thank my ex-wife, Kim; my late son, Rockson; my daughters Kauan and Kaulin; and my son, Kron, for their love and support, especially in the Tokyo Dome.

ACKNOWLEDGMENTS

I am grateful to my friend Sergio Zveiter for his wise counsel. I would also like to thank my old friends Bruce Weber, Susumu Nagao, and Marcos Prado for allowing me to use their photographs. I would like to thank Jocko Willink for writing the foreword. Last but not least, I want to thank my old friend and student Peter Maguire for helping me write this book and teaching me things about myself and the American side of my family that I did not know.

GLOSSARY OF TERMS

AMERICANA: A submission in which you grasp your opponent's wrist with one hand, bring your other arm underneath theirs, and grab your own wrist. With the opponent's elbow facing downward, you then use your grip to simultaneously push their wrist back and lift their elbow up. Also known as keylock, bent armlock, turkey bar, and *ude garami*.

ARM BAR: A lock in which the elbow joint is hyperextended. Also known as an armlock.

BASE: Refers to balance. Someone who is difficult to throw or sweep is described as having a "a good base."

BELTS: In Jiu Jitsu, there are five belts: white (*branca*), blue (*azul*), purple (*roxa*), brown (*marrom*), black (*preta*), coral (*cor coral*), and red (*vermelho/vermelha*).

BRIDGE: See UPA.

CHOKE: A submission hold applied to the neck that restricts the carotid arteries' blood flow to the brain.

CHOKE OUT: To choke an opponent unconscious.

CLINCH: A position in which one person holds another, either under or over their arms. In Jiu Jitsu, a clinch is often the prelude to a takedown.

CRANK: Unlike an arm bar, which must be precise, a crank is any move that uses force to wrench part of an opponent's body into an unnatural position to inflict pain. Because of the risk of serious injury, especially to the neck and spine, cranks are often banned and considered unsportsmanlike in Brazilian Jiu Jitsu circles.

ESCAPE: Any move by which one combatant gets out of a submission hold or other disadvantageous position.

GI: A heavy cotton uniform that consists of a pair of pants, a jacket, and a belt and is used by Judo and Jiu Jitsu practitioners.

GROUND AND POUND: A fighting technique pioneered by wrestlers who lacked submission skills so as to combat Jiu Jitsu in early MMA matches. Wrestlers would take their opponents to the ground, remain on top, and deliver strikes from either the guard, side control, or the mount.

GUARD: A position in which, while on your back, you wrap your legs around your opponent's torso. It can be used for both offense and defense.

GUILLOTINE: A choke applied by trapping your opponent's head and neck under your armpit, placing one forearm under the neck, grabbing your own wrist from the other side, and pulling upward. Successfully done, the move generates tremendous pressure.

HEEL: A professional wrestling villain.

HOOKS: Moves in which you take the back of your opponent and use your feet to control their legs so they can't turn and get you off their back.

JAB: A fast, lead-hand punch that is often used to soften up an opponent and set up a more powerful punch.

KIMURA: An armlock in which a victim's arm is twisted behind their back, breaking the arm or dislocating the shoulder if the fighter doesn't tap out. It was named after Japanese athlete Masahiko Kimura after he performed it on Hélio Gracie.

KNOCKOUT: The act of knocking one's opponent unconscious with a strike (a kick or punch).

MOUNT: A dominant Jiu Jitsu position in which you sit on top of your opponent with your legs straddling their torso.

NO-GI: Training without a gi jacket, often replacing the gi pants with shorts.

PASSING THE GUARD: The process of escaping from an opponent's guard and moving to side control, mount, or half guard.

PUNCH (HOOK): A loopy bent arm punch that strikes the opponent from the side.

PUNCH (STRAIGHT): A precise power punch thrown with the strong hand.

PUNCH (UPPERCUT): A bent-arm punch thrown straight up, often hitting the victim under the jaw.

REAR NAKED CHOKE: An arm choke that is applied from an opponent's back. Also known as *mata leão* ("to kill the lion" in Portuguese), *hadaka jime*, or sleeper hold.

ROLLING: A term often used in Jiu Jitsu and other grappling styles to mean sparring. When rolling, opponents attempt to submit each other.

SIDE CONTROL: A position in which you are on top but perpendicular to your opponent. Also known as side mount and cross-side.

SLAM: The act of picking one's opponent up and throwing them to the ground, sometimes knocking them out.

SPRAWL: A takedown defense wherein you spread your legs and drop your hips away from your attacker so as to deny them access to your legs and attain a superior position.

SUBMISSION: Any hold that forces an opponent to tap out, or renders an opponent injured or unconscious.

SWEEP: Any of numerous techniques in Jiu Jitsu that enable the person on the bottom to reverse an opponent and end up on top—e.g., scissor sweep.

TAKEDOWN: Any technique that takes an opponent down to the ground—a throw or a trip, for example.

TAKEDOWN (DOUBLE-LEG): As in a tackle, you lower your head, hook both of your opponent's legs behind the knees with your arms, and apply pressure to the upper body, driving your opponent to the ground.

TAKEDOWN (SINGLE-LEG): Similar to a double-leg takedown, except only one leg is grasped with the arms.

TAKE THE BACK: To secure a position on the back of one's opponent, aiming to get your legs wrapped around the hips, with your feet acting as hooks.

TAP, TAPPING: The act of slapping the ground, floor, or mat with your hand to indicate that you wish to concede—due to the pain of a submission hold or out of exhaustion. Sometimes people tap their opponent's body instead, or even use their feet if both arms are trapped.

TRIANGLE CHOKE: This choke is applied using the legs around your opponent's neck.

UFC: UFC (Ultimate Fighting Championship) is the biggest brand in combat sports and the driving force behind modern MMA (Mixed Martial Arts).

UNDERHOOK: Any position in which you get one of your limbs underneath one of your opponent's, such as under an arm when in the clinch.

UPA: Raising the hips when on your back, normally in an attempt to make space from under mount, but the move can also be used as part of other escapes. Also known as bridging.

WORK: As a noun, a fight with a prearranged outcome, also known as a "fixed" fight.

ABOUT THE AUTHORS

RICKSON GRACIE reigned as world Jiu Jitsu champion in both the middle-heavyweight and open divisions for almost two decades, retiring with an undefeated record after hundreds of Jiu Jitsu, *vale tudo*, and challenge matches. Since retiring, he has focused on unifying the Jiu Jitsu community and spreading his family martial art through his Jiu Jitsu Global Federation, teaching seminars around the world. A film about his life, *Dead or Alive*, directed by *Narcos* director José Padilha, is currently in development with Netflix.

PETER MAGUIRE is a military historian, journalist, and former war crimes investigator. He is the author of *Law and War*, *Facing Death in Cambodia*, and *Thai Stick*. Maguire has been Rickson Gracie's student and friend for more than twenty-five years, and is a coauthor of the script for the Rickson Gracie biopic, *Dead or Alive*.